ROBERT P. MATHIEU, M.S., F.A.C.H.A., F.A.P.H.A.

Administrator, Dr. U. E. Zambarano Memorial Hospital,
Wallum Lake, Rhode Island; Director, Division of Hospitals,
State of Rhode Island, Formerly Administrator,
Charles V. Chapin Hospital, Providence, Rhode Island

1971

W. B. SAUNDERS COMPANY

PHILADELPHIA · LONDON · TORONTO

HOSPITAL and NURSING HOME MANAGEMENT
an instructional and administrative manual

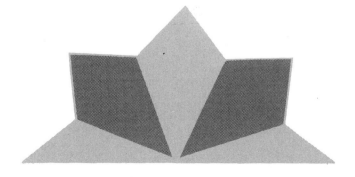

W. B. Saunders Company: West Washington Square
                           Philadelphia, Pa.   19105

                           12 Dyott Street
                           London, WC1A   1DB

                           1835 Yonge Street
                           Toronto 7, Ontario

Hospital and Nursing Home Management: an Instructional
    and Administrative Manual   SBN 0-7216-6188-2

Print No: 9   8   7   6   5   4   3   2   1

INTRODUCTION

This manual is designed for the purpose of guiding the health care facility administrator in the effective discharge of his responsibility — to provide a clean, healthy environment within which to protect and promote the health, safety and well-being of its patients. All physical, biological and social characteristics of the environment that influence the facets of good management are discussed in the pages that follow. The medical, administrative and fiscal aspects of the operation are also documented.

The material in this manual is a source of reference and an aid in the day to day administration of the facility. Numerous sections deal in detail with policies, procedures and practices necessary to the operation. Other sections, however, cover general policies and procedures because of the many differences in state and local laws, rules and regulations, differences in design and construction and even differences in types and levels of needs among patients served.

The administrator must be constantly alert to all the factors of environment and patient care involved as well as changes in emphasis dictated by government, medical practice and other external and internal influences. These require adjustment, augmentation and supplementation in line with the ever-changing needs of patients.

With this in mind, this manual attempts to provide the basic tools to enable you to perform your task in a manner satisfactory to yourself and your patients.

You are about to embark upon a very vital and humane venture. Dedication to this task and devotion to its duties will determine your success.

ROBERT P. MATHIEU

CONTENTS

Chapter 1
GENERAL REQUIREMENTS FOR THE EXTENDED CARE FACILITY 1

Chapter 2
PERSONNEL POLICIES 5

Chapter 3
PATIENT CARE POLICIES 17

Chapter 4
POLICIES ON PHYSICIANS' SERVICES 24

Chapter 5
NURSING SERVICE POLICIES 28

Chapter 6
DIETARY SERVICES 50

Chapter 7
RESTORATIVE SERVICES 94

Chapter 8
PHARMACEUTICALS—DISPENSING PROCEDURES 109

Chapter 9
DIAGNOSTIC, DENTAL AND PODIATRIC SERVICES 113

CHAPTER 10
SOCIAL SERVICES.. 115

CHAPTER 11
PATIENT ACTIVITIES... 119

CHAPTER 12
CLINICAL RECORDS.. 124

CHAPTER 13
TRANSFER AGREEMENTS... 167

CHAPTER 14
PHYSICAL ENVIRONMENT.. 181

CHAPTER 15
HOUSEKEEPING SERVICES.. 210

CHAPTER 16
LAUNDRY SERVICES 216

CHAPTER 17
DISASTER PLAN... 224

CHAPTER 18
ACCIDENT PREVENTION 227

CHAPTER 19
FIRE SAFETY 231

CHAPTER 20
BARBER AND BEAUTICIAN SERVICES.................................. 236

CHAPTER 21
UTILIZATION REVIEW PLAN 239

CHAPTER 22
BUSINESS SERVICES 244

CHAPTER 23
ACCREDITATION.. 266

INDEX 275

CHAPTER ONE

GENERAL REQUIREMENTS FOR THE EXTENDED CARE FACILITY

In order to participate as an extended care facility in the health insurance program for the aged, an institution must qualify within the requirements of section 1861 (j) of the Social Security Act, to wit:

FEDERAL STATUTORY REQUIREMENTS

An extended care facility must be an institution which has a transfer agreement with one or more hospitals and which is primarily engaged in providing to inpatients

1. Skilled nursing care and related services for patients who require medical or nursing care, or

2. Rehabilitation services for the rehabilitation of injured, disabled or sick persons.

Has policies developed and periodically reviewed by a professional group, including physicians and registered nurses, to govern the nursing care, related medicine or service it provides.

Has a physician, registered nurse or medical staff responsible for execution of such policies.

Has every patient under the supervision of a physician, and a physician available in case of emergency.

Maintains clinical records on all patients.

Provides 24 hour nursing sufficient to meet needs and has at least one registered nurse employed full time.

Provides appropriate methods and procedures for dispensing and administering drugs and biologicals.

Has a utilization review plan which meets the requirements.

Is licensed pursuant to any state or applicable local law and is approved by the respective agency of state or locality as meeting the standards for such licensing.

Meets such other conditions as the Secretary of Health, Education, and Welfare may impose.

These requirements briefly delineate the overall conditions of participation.

COMPLIANCE WITH STATE AND LOCAL LAWS

FACILITY LICENSE

The extended care facility shall comply with all applicable state or local laws for licensing of the facility.

It shall be licensed pursuant to such law.

It shall be approved by the agency of the State or locality responsible for licensing such institutions as meeting the standards established for such licensing.

STAFF LICENSE

All professional members of the staff shall be licensed or registered in accordance with applicable laws.

CONFORMITY WITH OTHER LAWS

This facility shall be in conformity with the laws relating to fire and safety, communicable and reportable diseases and any other applicable laws.

ADMINISTRATIVE MANAGEMENT

Governing Authority

The ownership of this facility shall be fully disclosed to the applicable state agency.

This ownership authority is responsible for compliance with applicable laws and regulations of legally authorized agencies.

Administration

This facility must have a full time administrator who is at least 21 years old, is capable of making mature judgments and has no physical or mental disabilities that interfere with carrying out his responsibilities.

The administrator has a minimum of a high school education and has had a reasonable amount of experience in the health field.

The administrator is responsible for the procurement and direction of competent personnel.

There is an individual competent and authorized to act in the absence of the administrator.

The administrative consultant and administrative physician are available to aid and assist the administration.

A full time administrative secretary is engaged.

Personnel Policies

Current employee records are maintained and include a resumé of each employee's training and experience.

The personnel file contains evidence of adequate health supervision, including results of pre-employment and periodic physical examinations, such as chest X-rays, and records of illnesses and accidents occurring while on duty.

All work assignments are consistent with employee qualifications.

Changes in Patient Status

This facility has approriate written policies and procedures relating to notification to responsible persons in the event of significant change in the patient's status, patient charges, billings and other related administrative matters.

Patients shall not be transferred or discharged without prior notification of next of kin or sponsors.

Information describing the care and services provided by the facility must be accurate and not misleading.

ADMINISTRATIVE CONSULTANT

Qualifications

The Administrative Consultant should preferably have a graduate degree in hospital administration from an accredited college. The consultant should have had at least five years of experience at the administrative level in the field of hospital administration. Furthermore he should currently be in the field, preferably in the position of administrator of a hospital.

Duties

The Administrative Consultant should be the liaison to the administrator of the facility. His duties should include advising the administrator and should further include observation of the operation of the facility. The consultant should regularly report his findings to the administrator and also suggest that corrective actions, where necessary, be taken.

ADMINISTRATIVE PHYSICIAN

Qualifications

The Administrative Physician should be a duly licensed physician in the particular state where the facility is located.

Duties

The Administrative Physician should aid and assist the administrator by participating in policies that affect the practice of medicine in the facility. He should function as the facility's physician and should attend all patients not under the care of a private attending physician. The Administrative Physician should further regularly review the care rendered to patients in the facility and evaluate the qualifications of the attending physicians.

ADMINISTRATIVE SECRETARY

The Administrative Secretary should be proficient in stenography as well as experienced in the responsibilities of handling routine administrative matters in behalf of the administrator.

Qualifications

Graduate of a business or secretarial college and/or a minimum of five years experience in a high level, executive secretarial position, preferably in the health field.

Able to take dictation proficiently and type with speed, accuracy and knowledge of procedure and format.

Able to capably represent administration in the use of the telephone and in the mechanics of communication, including letter and report writing.

Should be honest, dependable and presentable in appearance and personality.

Should be able to exert initiative and direction in fulfilling daily responsibilities.

Should be experienced in the diplomacy of dealing with members of the professions as well as with patients, families and other visitors.

Duties

The Administrative Secretary should function as the recording secretary for the minutes of all committees required in the operation of the facility.

Coordinate all of the reports from the various department heads, including the proper reporting to the insurance carrier and all accident and incident reports on patients and personnel.

Complete and maintain personnel folders on all personnel.

Coordinate the necessary requirements for all personnel with the local public health agency.

Insure that all stenographic and office supplies are available, including report forms and medical record forms.

Provide all confidential clerical work, including correspondence for the administrator.

Give initiative and judgment to routine matters, including correspondence and minor responsibilities of daily operation.

CHAPTER TWO

PERSONNEL POLICIES

The objective of the facility is to provide the best possible care to all patients by a staff who are trained in and demonstrate the willingness to give of themselves and their abilities to patient care. These personnel policies are intended to explain the positions of both administration and personnel in relation to their duties.

RESPONSIBILITIES OF ADMINISTRATION

The administration should employ only those personnel qualified to perform their duties and should assure by orientation and in-service education, if necessary, that only qualified personnel are accepted. Training programs should be provided in order to allow for promotion of personnel who have demonstrated these qualifications.

Salaries competitive with those of similar facilities in the area as well as good working conditions and security of employment should be assured all personnel.

The facility should strive to maintain good working relations with all personnel and must see to it that discrimination of any nature is not allowed.

RESPONSIBILITIES OF PERSONNEL

ABSENTEEISM

All personnel must notify their immediate supervisor not less than one-half hour prior to their time of reporting for work if for any reason they are unable to report.

In the event of death or serious emergency in the immediate family of personnel, absence with pay may be allowed at the discretion of the administrator.

Extended leaves of absence shall be considered and may be granted with or without pay whenever the need appears justified by the administrator.

ACCIDENTS OR INJURIES ON THE JOB

All accidents and injuries must be reported at once to the immediate supervisor. The proper reporting form should be completed and forwarded to the office of the administrator.

CHANGE OF ADDRESS OR STATUS

All personnel must provide the business office of the facility with current address, marital status, telephone number and other pertinent information in connection with these matters.

PERSONNEL APPEARANCE AND GROOMING

Good grooming, cleanliness, neatness and personal hygiene habits are necessary for all personnel.

INFORMATION BOARD

Official information and bulletin boards should be located in convenient locations by department for all personnel. Information on these boards is restricted to official information from administration and should apply to all personnel.

PERSONNEL SOLICITING

Solicitation of any kind for whatever purpose, including ticket selling or merchandising by personnel or others, is strictly prohibited.

STANDARDS OF CONDUCT

All personnel are expected to maintain the highest standards of conduct. Proper respect toward patients, visitors and fellow personnel must be maintained. All conduct including unnecessary noise and talk and other activities that are found to be disturbing to patients and other personnel must be avoided. All information regarding patients is privileged information and is confidential and therefore is not allowed to be transmitted to anyone without authority from administration.

PERSONNEL CREDIT CHARACTER

All personnel should be cautioned to plan their credit standards in such a manner that the facility is not involved in a garnishment of wages. Such involvement may be grounds for dismissal.

CONDITIONS OF EMPLOYMENT

All personnel should be urged to freely discuss with their immediate supervisor all matters affecting their employment. Any matters not resolved at this level may be referred to the administrator for further consideration.

SAFETY AND FIRE RULES

Safety rules and fire regulations are posted on all information bulletin boards. All personnel are expected to familiarize themselves with these regulations and understand their precise role in any emergency. All personnel are requested to report any conditions that they feel are fire and accident prone in nature. Smoking by personnel is allowed only in those areas specifically designated for this purpose.

GRATUITIES

Personnel are prohibited from accepting gratuities of any kind, including tips, or gifts from patients, visitors or other personnel.

PERSONNEL HEALTH

In order to assure good health of all personnel it is necessary for each to have a physical examination and chest x-ray upon employment and at subsequent times during employment when required by health authorities and when considered in the best interests of personnel and the facility.

HOLY DAYS—RELIGIOUS HOLIDAYS

Special holy days or specific religious holidays may be observed by those personnel wishing to do so by special request through the immediate supervisor. Absence from duty for these purposes may be charged against vacation time.

HOSPITAL HEALTH CLINIC

All personnel injured or ill while on duty will be given health treatment within the facility. This treatment must be restricted to that of an emergency nature and any prolonged treatment or hospitalization shall be the responsibility of the individual.

LOITERING

All personnel are required to leave their place of employment immediately on the completion of their duties in order to prevent confusion and interference with the work schedule.

LOST AND FOUND

The administration cannot accept the responsibility for articles lost or stolen within the facility by personnel. All personnel must be responsible to safeguard the property of others as well as their own. This should include the return of any found property to its owner. Any articles found within the facility may be turned over to the office of the administrator for identification and return to the owner.

MAIL

Personnel are not allowed to use the address of the facility for the conduct of personal correspondence by mail.

PROMOTIONS

It is the policy of the facility to promote from within. Preference and promotions are given to current personnel on the basis of seniority, past performance, qualifications and abilities.

DESTRUCTION OF PROPERTY

Negligence on the part of all personnel resulting in destruction of facility property should be accounted for. The facility's name or other property may not at any time be used by any personnel for their own personal benefit.

SALARY

All personnel are made fully aware of salary and deductions upon employment. Checks are issued on a regularly scheduled basis. All salary increases are effective at the beginning of the respective month.

TELEPHONE

Personnel may not use the official business telephones of the facility for personal business, except in case of serious emergency. Public telephones are available for personal calls.

TERMINATION

All personnel are requested to provide two weeks of notice prior to voluntary termination of employment.

Termination of employment notice on the part of the administration also provides two weeks of notice to all personnel, except in the case of dismissal, wherein no notice is necessary and personnel may be separated immediately.

TRAINING PROGRAMS

In-service training programs are available and must be participated in by all personnel within their areas of duty.

UNIFORMS

Any uniforms required by virtue of profession or nature of duties are the responsibility of personnel for purchase and satisfactory maintenance.

VACATIONS

A regular schedule of vacation allowance is provided for all full time personnel and is established on the basis of years of service rendered.

WORKMEN'S COMPENSATION—SOCIAL SECURITY

All personnel are included in the provisions of the Workmen's Compensation Act and are protected under the Federal Social Security Program.

WORK HOURS—PERFORMANCE

The day shift is designed to begin at 7:00 A.M. and end at 3:30 P.M., allowing one-half hour for lunch.

The evening shift begins at 3:00 P.M. and extends to 11:30 P.M., allowing for one-half hour for supper.

The night shift extends from 11:00 P.M. to 7:00 A.M., with time for a meal allowed on work time.

Brief rest periods may be allowed in all departments under the authority of the immediate supervisors.

Personnel are not allowed to leave their places of employment without permission during their regular working hours.

Performance of duty forms shall be completed on all personnel by their immediate supervisors. These reports will be reviewed by the administration on a regular basis.

APPLICATION FOR EMPLOYMENT

Mr.
Mrs.
NAME Miss _____   Social
            Last   First   Initial   Security No. _____

ADDRESS _____   PHONE _____
            Street & Number   City   State

NEAREST   ☐ Wife   RELATIVE'S
RELATIVE _____   ☐ Husband   ADDRESS _____
                           ☐ Other

BIRTHDATE _____   MARITAL   Married   Widowed   Professional
            Mo. Day Year STATUS   Single   Divorced   License No. _____ Type _____

NUMBER OF _____ OVER 18
CHILDREN _____ UNDER 18   OTHER DEPENDENTS _____
                                         What relationship to you?

TYPE WORK   WAGES
DESIRED _____   EXPECTED _____

| PREVIOUS WORK EXPERIENCE | | (List Last Employment First) | | |
DATE	EMPLOYER	SUPERVISOR	POSITION	REASON FOR LEAVING
FROM-	Name	Name	Title	
TO-	Address	Title	Salary	
FROM-	Name	Name	Title	
TO-	Address	Title	Salary	

RECEIVED PAYMENT		
UNEMPLOYMENT INSURANCE	WORKMEN'S COMPENSATION	DISABILITY INSURANCE
☐ YES ☐ NO	☐ YES ☐ NO	☐ YES ☐ NO
DATE	DATE	DATE

LAST SCHOOL _____   ☐ YES
                                                  ☐ NO
            Name   Grade   Vocation   Diploma

PHYSICAL INFORMATION			
HEIGHT WEIGHT CONDITION OF HEALTH	☐ EXCELLENT	☐ GOOD	☐ POOR
HAVE YOU EVER HAD TROUBLE WITH? HEART	LUNGS		HERNIA
ANY DEFECTS IN? SPEECH	SIGHT	HEARING	BACK
OTHER AILMENTS OR DISABILITIES(SUCH AS ASTHMA,SINUS,BACKACHES,ETC.). LIST:			

| CHARACTER REFERENCES   (| Persons Who Know You Well. | |) | | |
	(Do not include relatives or employees.)				
NAME	OCCUPATION	STREET	CITY	STATE	YEARS KNOWN
(1)					
(2)					
(3)					

   I certify that all statements made in this application are, to the best of my knowledge,
correct. Should any of the statements be subsequently proved inaccurate, I understand the employer may cancel any employment agreement made with me. You have permission to contact my
previous employers.

   DATE _____   SIGNED _____

APPLICATION FOR EMPLOYMENT — *Continued*

NAME

EVALUATION AND RESULT OF APPLICATION

INTERVIEWER'S ESTIMATE: ☐ DESIRABLE   ☐ CHECK EMPLOYERS   ☐ NOT SUITABLE

REFERENCES' ESTIMATE: ☐ STRONGLY FAVORABLE ☐ MODERATELY FAVORABLE   ☐ ROUTINE
☐ NEGATIVE   WHY?

ACCEPTED: JOB ASSIGNMENT   STARTING PAY $

DATE TO REPORT   DATE STARTED

REJECTED: ☐ KEEP FILE ACTIVE   ☐ POSSIBLE PROSPECT   ☐ DO NOT CONTACT FURTHER

PERIODIC EVALUATION OF EMPLOYEE

	FIRST MONTH	SIX MONTHS	FIRST YEAR	SECOND YEAR	THIRD YEAR
PROMPT					
DILIGENT					
COOPERATIVE					
RELIABLE					
QUALITY OF WORK					
COMMENTS					

EMPLOYMENT RECORD

JOB CHANGES DESCRIPTION	DATE	DATE	RATE	DATE	RATE	DATE	RATE
			$		$		$
			$		$		$

TIME AWAY FROM JOB

VACATION DATE	DATE	SICK LEAVE	ABSENT	TIME OFF	EXPLANATION

TERMINATION OF EMPLOYMENT

DATE OF TERMINATION:

BASIS OF TERMINATION:

CONFIDENTIAL: SHOULD EMPLOYEE BE RECOMMENDED?
SHOULD EMPLOYEE BE RE-HIRED IF APPLYING?

LAST CHECK: $ Amount   Date   Check Number   Date Paid

CLAIMS DUE (EXPLAIN):

MAILING ADDRESS:

APPLICATION FOR EMPLOYMENT—*Continued*

Name_____ Soc.Sec.
Number_____ Date_____ 19_____

Address_____Phone_____

Position Applied for_____

In case of emergency notify_____Relationship_____

Address_____Phone_____

Date of Birth_____ Where Born_____Citizen of_____

Religion_____ Single___ Married___ Widowed___ Divorced___ No.of Dependents___

Basic education	and RECENT Continuing education					
Name and Location of Schools or Colleges	Major Subject	Did you Graduate	College Degree	Period of Attendance From	To

FORMER EMPLOYERS AND EXPERIENCE (References)						
Name and Address	Nature of Experience	Period From	To	Cash Salary	Other Compensations	Reason for Leaving

PERSONAL REFERENCES (Not relatives)			
NAME	ADDRESS	PHONE	BUSINESS

HEALTH   RECORD

1. Do you have any physical limitations that should be considered?_____
   If answer is yes, describe:_____

2. List name and address of your personal physician._____

3. Give date and place of last general physical checkup._____

4. Have you ever filed a claim under Workman's Compensation Act?_____
   If so, what year?_____ Where?_____ Under what circumstances?_____

5. Were you ever hospitalized for injury or illness?____ Give details-year,name of hospital,
   location of hospital,etc._____

WORK PERFORMANCE REPORT

Personnel _____   Date _____

Immediate Supervisor _____

Below Aver.	Aver.	Above Aver.	
___	___	___	Reports on time
___	___	___	Absenteeism
___	___	___	Attendance
___	___	___	Reports occurrences
___	___	___	Performs tasks efficiently
___	___	___	Uses good judgment
___	___	___	Loyalty and pride to duty
___	___	___	Understands job requirements
___	___	___	Considers the religious preferences of the patient
___	___	___	Has positive attitude toward patient
___	___	___	Cooperates with supervisor
___	___	___	Cooperates with personnel
___	___	___	Discharge of duties
___	___	___	Leadership ability
___	___	___	Has the ability to act independently
___	___	___	Seeks help and guidance when needed
___	___	___	Seeks knowledge for job performance
___	___	___	Knowledge of procedures, policies, and understanding of fire and disaster plan
___	___	___	Attentive to notices
___	___	___	Participates
___	___	___	Accepts constructive criticism
___	___	___	Attends meetings
___	___	___	Shows evidence of learning from experience and instruction
___	___	___	Uses equipment properly
___	___	___	Appreciates value of equipment
___	___	___	Assumes responsibility
___	___	___	Friendly
___	___	___	Good moral character
___	___	___	Cooperative

Signature of Immediate Supervisor   _____

Signature of personnel testifying to knowledge of rating _____

RECORDING OF WORK TIME

All personnel must report to their immediate supervisor at the beginning of their work day. Promptness in reporting for work is essential. All patterns of tardiness are to be noted by the immediate supervisor; continuous infractions may be grounds for dismissal.

All personnel must personally sign in and out. No one may sign for any fellow employee under any conditions.

SEVEN-WEEK CYCLE, STRAIGHT-SHIFT PLAN

Seven-Week Cycle, Straight-Shift Plan

Nurse (or team) No.	1st Week m t w t f s s	2nd Week m t w t f s s	3rd Week m t w t f s s	4th Week m t w t f s s	5th Week m t w t f s s	6th Week m t w t f s s	7th Week m t w t f s s
1 8	x x x x x	x x x x x	x x x x x	x x x x x	x x x x x x	x x x x x x	x x x x x
2 9	x x x x	x x x x x	x x x x x x	x x x x x x	x x x x x	x x x x x	x x x x x x
3 10 etc.	x x x x x	x x x x x	x x x x x	x x x x x x	x x x x x	x x x x x x	x x x x x x
4	x x x x x	x x x x	x x x x x x	x x x x x x	x x x x x	x x x x x	x x x x x x
5	x x x x x	x x x x x	x x x x x x	x x x x x	x x x x x x	x x x x	x x x x x x
6	x x x	x x x x x	x x x x	x x x x x x	x x x x x x	x x x x x	x x x x x x
7	x x x	x x x x x	x x x x x	x x x x x x	x x x x x	x x x x	x x x x x x

Twenty-Week Cycle, Rotating-Shift Plan

Nurse (or team) No.	1st Week m t w t f s s	2nd Week m t w t f s s	3rd Week m t w t f s s	4th Week m t w t f s s	5th Week m t w t f s s	6th Week m t w t f s s	7th Week m t·w t f s s
1	d d d d	d d d d d	n n n n	d d d d	e e e e n n	n n n d d	d d d
2	n n d d	e e e e	e e e n n n	n n d d d	n n d d d d	e e n n n n	n d d d
3	e n n n n	d d d d d	e e e e	e n n n n	d d d e e e e	d d d d	n n n n n
4	e e e e e	n n n n	d d d d d	e e e e e	n n n n n	d d d d d	e e e e n

Nurse (or team) No.	8th Week m t w t f s s	9th Week m t w t f s s	10th Week m t w t f s s	11th Week m t w t f s s	12th Week m t w t f s s	13th Week m t w t f s s	14th Week m t w t f s s
1	e e e n n n	n n d d d d	d d e e e	e e n n n n n	n d d d d	d e e e e	e n n n n n
2	d e e e e	e n n n n n	d d d d	d d d d	n n n n d d	d d d d	e e e e
3	d d d d	e e e e	n n n n n	e e e e	e e e e	n n n d d d	d d d d d d d
4	n n n n d	d d d d e	e e e e n n	n n n d d	d d d e e	e e e n n n	n n d d d

Nurse (or team) No.	15th Week m t w t f s s	16th Week m t w t f s s	17th Week m t w t f s s	18th Week m t w t f s s	19th Week m t w t f s s	20th Week m t w t f s s	21st Week
1	d d d d d	e e e e e	n n n n n	d d d d d	e e e e e	n n n n n	
2	n n n n n	d d d d d	e e e e	n n n n d	e e e e	e e e n n	
3	e e e n n	d d e e e e	e e e n n	d d d d e	d d d e e	d d e e e	
4	d d e e e	e e n n n n	n n d d d d	e e e n n	e e e n n n	d d d d d	

Four-Week Cycle, Rotating-Shift Plan

Nurse (or team) No.	m t w t f s s	m t w t f s s	m t w t f s s	m t w t f s s
1	n n n n n	d d d d d d	e e e e e	n n n
2	e e e n n	n n n n n	d d d d d	e e e e
3	d e e e e	e e e n n	n n n n n	d d d d d
4	d d d d d	d e e e e	e e e n n	n n n n n

d = Day Shift   e = Evening Shift   n = Night Shift

SEVEN-WEEK CYCLE, STRAIGHT SHIFT PLAN—*Continued*

Seven-Week Cycle, Alternating-Shift Plan

Nurse (or Team) No.	1st Week m t w t f* s s	2nd Week m t w t f s s*	3rd Week m t w t f s s*	4th Week m* t w t f s s	5th Week m t* w t f s s	6th Week m t w* t f s s	7th Week m t w t* f s s
1	d d d d d	e e e e e	d d d d d	e e e e e	e e d d d	d d d e e e	e e d d d
2	e e e d d d d	d d d d d e e	d d d e e e	e e d d d d d	d d d e e e e	d d d d e e e	e e e d d d d
3	e e d d d d d	d d d e e e e	d d e e e e	d d d d e e e	e e e d d d d	d d d d d	d e e e

d = Day shift   e = Evening Shift   n = Night Shift   * = Extra nurse available for relief duty.

ACCIDENT OR INCIDENT REPORT
(Report all accidents or incidents even if no apparent injury)

Family Name   First Name   Middle Name   Room No.   Bed No.   Admission No.

a.m.

Date of accident or incident _____19___Time_____p.m.   Place_____

a.m.

Was it necessary to notify physican?   yes___ no___Time of notification_____p.m.

Name of Physician _____ Name of supervision nurse_____

Describe nature of accident or incident and injuries received: _____

_____

_____

_____

_____

_____

_____

_____

_____

_____

a.m.

Date of written report _____ 19 _____Time_____p.m.

Signed _____
Physician or Nurse

CHAPTER THREE

PATIENT CARE POLICIES

REQUIREMENTS

Title XVIII—Extended Care Facility:

"There are policies to govern the skilled nursing care and related medical or other services provided, which are developed with the advice of professional personnel, including one or more physicians and one or more registered professional nurses. A physician, a registered professional nurse, or a medical staff is responsible for the execution of these policies."

Title XIX—Skilled Nursing Home:

"Patient care is provided in accordance with written policies formulated with the advice of one or more physicians and one or more registered professional nurses."

Joint Commission on Accreditation of Hospitals—
Nursing Care Facility and Residential Care Facility:

"There shall be evidence in writing of acceptable administrative policies, practices, and procedures. There shall be a prepared administrative manual explaining patient/resident care policies and procedures in regard to admissions, discharges, refunds, and other pertinent information relating to the total operation of the facility. Responsible persons shall be informed periodically regarding the condition of the patient/resident and notified in the event of an emergency change in patient/resident status."

"There shall be two (2) or more duly licensed doctors of medicine who shall agree in writing to advise on medical-administrative problems, review the institution's program of patient care, provide for utilization review, and handle emergencies if the individual's personal physician is unavailable."

ORGANIZATION CHART

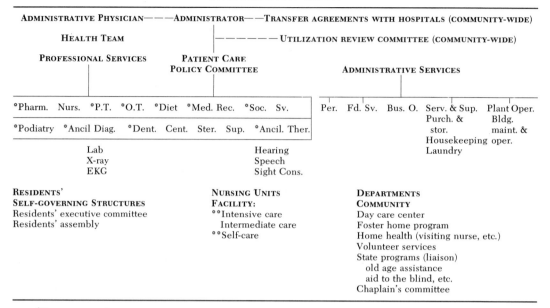

°By arrangements.

°°Under "distinct part" provisions of Titles XVIII and XIX (Consultation services offered by health professionals from the community).

PATIENT CARE POLICY COMMITTEE

To organize and maintain effective patient care, a patient care policy committee should be established. Following is the proposed form for an agreement to establish such a committee.

Date Adopted ——————————

Foreword

Recognizing that the patient care policy committee is responsible for the quality of medical care in the facility, and must accept and assume this responsibility, subject to the ultimate authority of the ownership, and that the best interests of the patient are protected by concerted effort, the physicians, dentists, and health professionals practicing and offering their services to patients in the facility hereby organize themselves in conformity with this statement of organization. For the purpose of this statement of organization, the words "medical staff" shall be interpreted to include all physicians and dentists who are privileged to attend patients in the facility.

Organization

Name

The name of this organization shall be the patient care policy committee.

Purpose

The purposes of this committee shall be as follows:

To insure that all patients admitted to the facility receive the best possible care.

To provide a means whereby problems of a medical-administrative nature may be considered by the committee.

To establish, execute and review patient care policies on medical, dental and nursing service practices in the facility.

To provide education and to maintain educational standards.

To provide advice and recommendations to the ownership and to the medical director and administrative physician on medical and administrative matters affecting the facility.

Treatment goals for patients

The efforts of this patient care policy committee will be directed toward effecting staff effort (including the full range of the community's health and social services) toward accomplishment of the following goals for patients.

To achieve and maintain their maximum potentials;

To develop latent interests and capabilities;

To regain the ability to develop interpersonal relationships; and

To orient toward living outside the facility, when feasible.

Committee membership

The membership of this committee shall be composed of physicians, dentists or health practitioners who serve the health and social needs of patients in this facility as staff members, full- or part-time, or as consultants or advisors to the staff, and who meet these qualifications:

A physician or dentist shall be of good character, legally licensed to practice medicine or dentistry in the State of _____, a staff member or eligible for staff membership in a recognized hospital and practicing within a reasonable distance of this facility.

A health practitioner shall have completed the required academic preparation in a health profession and is licensed or registered by a state authority or certified by an appropriate professional association.

MEDICAL DIRECTOR – ADMINISTRATIVE PHYSICIAN

One physician shall be designated as medical director–administrative physician. He shall be appointed by the ownership in cooperation with the administrator annually. He shall be responsible to the ownership and administrator. The medical director–administrative physician shall be an ex-officio member of all advisory committees of the patient care policy committee.

The medical director–administrative physician shall help to develop medical and patient care policies concerning patient admission and discharge, medical records, physicians' responsibility for their patients and other matters concerning patient care. In clinical matters, he shall give guidance on restorative care (rehabilitation) programs, nursing procedures and in-service programs for nursing personnel. He shall be responsible for reviewing the qualifications of medical, dental and paramedical personnel who are employed or utilized or who otherwise attend to the needs of patients in the facility.

OFFICERS

The officers of the patient care policy committee shall be the chairman and secretary.

The chairman, who shall be the medical director–administrative physician, shall call and preside at all meetings, shall be a member ex-officio of all advisory committees and shall have general supervision over all the professional work of the committee. The chairman shall be appointed by the ownership annually after consultation with physicians and dentists, the administrator and the director of nursing service of the facility.

The secretary shall keep complete minutes of all meetings, call meetings on order of the chairman, attend to all correspondence and perform such other duties as ordinarily pertain to this office. He shall also act as treasurer (where committee funds are to be accounted for). The secretary shall be appointed by the ownership annually after consultation with the medical director–administrative physician and the administrator. The administrator should serve as secretary.

Functions of the committee

The committee shall establish the level(s) of care that the facility intends to provide, establish general policy, anticipate future needs and serve as a planning body. The general policies to be established shall include, among others, the following areas:

Admission, transfer and discharge policies, including categories of patients accepted and not accepted by the extended care facility

Physician services
Nursing services
Dietary services
Restorative (rehabilitation) services
Pharmaceutical services
Diagnostic services
Care of patients in an emergency, during a communicable disease episode and when critically ill or mentally disturbed
Dental services
Podiatric services
Social services
Patient activities
Clinical records
Transfer agreement
Utilization and medical review.

The committee shall be fully cognizant of the preparations that the facility has made to deliver the proposed level(s) of care as expressed in staffing patterns— availability of personnel with appropriate abilities, availability of equipment and sufficiency of the physical plant for use by personnel.

The committee shall make regular assessments of the manner in which the facility as an entity is carrying out its functions and shall recommend corrective actions to the ownership when the occasion demands. The committee shall accomplish its functions with the active assistance of several advisory committees.

Functions of the advisory committees

Three advisory committees shall be activated to assist the committee in the accomplishment of its responsibilities. The committee shall be the final determinant in all decisions recommended by the advisory committees and shall be responsible for corrective actions involving physicians, dentists and staff members.

THE PROGRAM ASSESSMENT ADVISORY COMMITTEE

The program assessment advisory committee shall make regular assessments of the manner in which the facility as an entity is carrying out its functions. These assessments will determine that reasonable precautions are being taken and will assure that physicians and personnel taking part in the care of the patient measure up to recognized standards. The advisory committee shall assure that each patient's health and social needs are being effectively met, that the expenditure of effort is producing the best possible results and that consideration is given to the feasibility of meeting these health care needs through alternative services.

This committee shall assist the utilization review committee and the medical review team in determining that the facility is promoting the most efficient use of available health facilities and services by identification and analysis of patterns of patient care.

THE MEDICAL RECORDS ADVISORY COMMITTEE

The medical records advisory committee shall regularly review the medical records by making a "quantitative audit" of each record and shall provide supervision and appraisal to insure their maintenance at the required standard. The medical record system will encompass basic and essential facts about the patient, beginning with the transfer or referral statement before the patient is admitted and extending to every aspect of his care until discharge and possible referral to a home health agency.

The committee shall provide essential information needed by the utilization review committee, the medical review team, and assist those groups in selection of cases for study.

THE PHARMACY AND THERAPEUTICS ADVISORY COMMITTEE

The pharmacy and therapeutics advisory committee shall work with the full- or part-time pharmacist to establish the proper administrative authority in the facility for developing, supervising and coordinating the activities of the pharmaceutical services to patients as the system relates to selection, evaluation and distribution of drugs used in the facility.

The administrator shall, in routinely participating in the work of the several advisory committees, offer assistance in formulating adequate and timely reports on their findings. The reports will be offered to the patient care policy committee so that its members may be assured that the staff of the facility is securing results which conform to approved standards and are in accordance with its policies.

The utilization review function

The utilization review and medical review functions will be accomplished by outside groups. The patient care policy committee will take every step to insure that the utilization review committee and medical review team have the support and assistance of the facility's administrative staff in assembling information, facilitating chart reviews, conducting studies, exploring ways to improve procedures, maintaining committee records and promoting the most efficient use of available health services and facilities, including alternative services.

Meetings

The patient care policy committee shall meet quarterly. At these meetings the advisory committees shall report to the patient care policy committee, and recommendations shall be made for reappointment of committee members.

Special meetings of the patient care policy committee may be called at any time by the chairman or at the request of two members of the committee, giving reasonable advance notice thereof to members.

Members of the patient care policy committee are expected to attend all meetings.

At each meeting the chairman shall present an analysis of the work of the facility during the previous quarter, and the meeting shall be devoted to a study of this analysis and a general review of the medical records. Insofar as the occurrence of cases of interest will allow, the members will rotate regularly in presenting cases for discussion.

The agenda shall be as follows:
1. Call to order
2. Reading of the minutes of the last regular and of all special meetings
3. Unfinished business
4. Communications
5. Reports of advisory committees
6. Review and analysis of the clinical work of the facility (by the medical director—administrative physician)
7. New business
8. Discussion and recommendations for improvement of the professional work of the facility
9. Administrator's report
10. Adjournment

Formulation of Procedures

The head of each department shall be required to submit in detail the procedures that can be standardized for his department. Any of these procedures that may affect another department shall then be submitted to the head of the second department and modified, if necessary, to smooth interdepartmental functioning.

Health practitioners who serve as consultants or part-time staff members shall be called upon to develop procedures which will affect their activities in the facility.

Subject to the approval of the patient care policy committee, the procedures will be issued by authority of the administrator.

The procedures shall be issued in a loose-leaf binder, a sufficient number being supplied to allow easy access for reference by all personnel of each department concerned. Master copies shall be issued to the chief administrative officers, and only those sections which apply to the individual departments will be distributed further.

The order of placement in the binder shall be, first, general procedures which affect two or more departments and, second, special orders which concern only the department to which they are issued. Procedures will be kept separate from standing orders (orders to all personnel which may be applicable to any patient).

A standard format for procedures shall be used by all departments.

Procedures shall include detail of all operations covering at least the areas listed.

Business procedures which do not affect the professional care of the patient shall also be developed in collaboration with the several members of the patient care policy committee. These will be subject to the approval of the ownership and likewise will be issued by authority of the administrator.

Amendments to statement of organization

The provisions of this statement of organization and functions of the patient care policy committee may be amended after notice at any regular meeting of the committee. Amendments so made shall be effective when approved by the ownership.

Adoption

This statement of organization shall be adopted by the committee and shall become effective when approved by the ownership.

Adopted by the patient care policy committee of the facility.

_____
Chairman

_____
Secretary

Date _____
Approved by the ownership

_____
Secretary of the Ownership

Date _____

THE PRIVILEGES OF PATIENTS, FAMILIES AND VISITORS

PATIENTS

It is the duty of the facility to provide all the care required for the comfort of the patient and necessary to his maximum restoration to good health.

The facility must also provide personnel qualified by virtue of their education and training to carry out the responsibilities to which they are assigned, including adequate nursing personnel who, by knowledge and sensitivity to the needs of the patient, service these needs with dispatch and feeling.

Under the authority of the attending physician the facility must provide social services to the patient regarding his illness in order that he and his family may best be able to understand and adjust to the illness.

The patient and his family should further be consulted in cases where more intensive services might be available in order that they may be knowledgeable of the patient's needs and able to cope with them.

It is the responsibility of all nursing personnel to respect the confidential nature of the patient's illness and all records which relate to the patient.

Every effort shall be made to make the patient's surroundings as pleasant and cheerful as possible in order for the patient to better accept his illness.

FAMILIES

Families have a right to expect that the total care of the patient will be provided in an efficient manner under the authority of a certified physician, and that all rights of the patient will be understood, respected and adhered to.

The proper authorities must provide continuing information regarding the condition of the patient. A total description of the nature of the patient's illness should be fully discussed with the family in order for them to better understand the nature of the patient's illness so that they can formulate their own evaluation of the overall care provided to the patient.

Families have a right to expect that all health care, restorative and rehabilitative services will be provided wherever and whenever it is possible in the best interests of the health of the patient, and that treatment to all patients will be provided strictly under the written order of the attending physician only.

Official visiting hours should be established and the proper visitors, including members of the immediate family and others authorized, be allowed to visit the patient. Particular visitors should not be excluded where there appears to be a dispute among members of the immediate family. Family disputes should be settled outside of the patient's setting. Alienation of patient's affections for a member of his family is a serious charge against any personnel; no members of the staff are allowed to enter into or arbitrate family disputes.

An official and effective change of condition formula should be available, and the family of a patient must be promptly notified when the condition of the patient becomes dangerous. The family should· be urged to be immediately available at the bedside when this is indicated.

No changes in the financial or service structure should be made without reasonable and prior notice to the family.

The patient's valuables are his property and should be turned over to the proper nearest of kin, as established by law, upon his demise.

VISITORS

Visiting should be established by policy as to hours and length of visit.

Food and snacks brought to the patient by visitors are allowed only in the amount that may be consumed during the period of the visit and only of a sort allowed by the attending physician.

No storage of foods should be allowed in the nursing unit refrigeration facilities.

Alcoholic beverages should never be permitted to be brought by visitors. The attending physician may order service of alcoholic beverage to patients for medicinal purposes, and these beverages must be provided only through the proper drug and nursing service.

Smoking should never be allowed in any areas of nursing service, particularly in patients' rooms. Patients who smoke may do so only under the immediate attention and direct authority of the nurse supervising the unit.

CHAPTER FOUR

POLICIES ON PHYSICIANS' SERVICES

RESPONSIBILITY

The responsibility of the physician is to provide the diagnosis and to recommend the course of care required for the needs of the patient in his illness, and should include orders for medicines and drugs, ancillary diagnostic services and any rehabilitative program required, as determined by examination and diagnosis.

ATTENDING AND ADMINISTRATIVE PHYSICIANS

The attending physician must be one duly licensed to practice medicine in the state (this includes duly licensed dentists). The attending physician is the one who has recommended the admission and has been provided the privilege of treating the patient.

The administrative physician must also be duly licensed to practice medicine in the state and is the one who is available to assure the proper care of the patient when the private attending physician is not available.

ADMISSION

Patients should be admitted only on specific recommendation of the referring physician. Requirements of the physician prior to admission include a pre-admission impression, a medical summary and physician's orders regarding the care and treatment of the patient. It is preferred that all admissions be made on a prescheduled basis. Those admissions allowed under urgent conditions must be made in such a manner that they include the immediate attention of the referring physician to assure safe and proper treatment of the patient.

All patients must have continuing attention and orders for treatment from a physician, be he the attending physician permitted or the administrative physician provided. In either case the physician must comply with the policies and procedures laid down regarding admission, treatment, medical records and all other medical matters pertinent to good patient care.

The indicated physician is responsible for the history taken and physical examination performed upon admission of the patient. In no case are these done more than 48 hours following admission.

ORDERS FOR SUPERVISION, MEDICATION AND TREATMENT

The patient's physician, only, is responsible for the doctor's orders for treatment and medicines and drugs and the proper recordings thereof in the medical record, attested to by his signature. All orders are effective for the number of days specified by the physician and no orders may be written for longer than a one month period, wherein reordering must be made in writing by the physician. In the case of an attending physician, when it is determined by the nursing supervision that his presence is necessary to the best interest of the patient, it is his responsibility to respond immediately or provide for covered services to assure proper attention to the needs of the patient. Where the attending physician fails to provide for this service, the administrative physician should assume immediate responsibility for the continuing care of the patient. The attending physician should be allowed to resume his responsibility only upon satisfactory explanation and assurance that he is prepared to carry out the responsibility effectively.

Telephone orders made by the attending physician may be accepted only by a licensed registered or practical nurse. Said nurse should enter the order in the patient's record on the doctor's order sheet and should be verified by telephone with the physician prior to carrying out the orders. The ordering physician must countersign such an entry within 24 hours.

The indicated physician must review the patient's medical record and the course of care provided the patient at regular intervals, and in no case should such interval exceed one month. Any revisions or changes in the program of care should be recorded in the progress notes and on the doctor's order sheet when indicated.

The physician must attend his patient with regularity. In no case should this visit interval exceed one month. In most cases the interval should be considerably more frequent. A quality progress note must be entered in the medical record. Failure on the part of the attending physician to provide this service will result in the administrative physician assuming this responsibility until such time as the attending physician is able to verify and certify his ability to resume attendance of the patient. In all cases the patient and the responsible nearest of kin will be notified of this action.

The social service sheet of the medical record should contain all necessary information regarding the schedule of the attending physician and the coverage he has provided himself during periods of absence from his practice. This information should contain the name, or names, and addresses and telephone numbers of the covering physicians in the order in which they should be called in his absence in the event of need by the patient.

Consultation from a qualified physician is the responsibility of the attending physician when necessary due to a question of diagnosis or doubt as to the proper care required by the patient. A descriptive request for consultation must be written by the attending physician in the medical record and the responsive consultation must include written verification of examination of the patient and the medical record and a written report recorded in the medical record signed by the consultant.

Physical restraints should be applied to patients only under the direct order of the attending physician. Close attention during periods of restraint must be given by the nursing service, with the intervals between immediate attention for safety of restraint being made not more than one half-hour during the patient's waking hours and not more than one hour during his hours of sleep.

Standing orders for all patients are a necessity and must be formulated by the administration and the administrative physician and confirmed with each attending physician on admission of his patient. Standing orders should be utilized only when specific orders in regards to the immediate need of the patient are not written by the attending physician.

EMERGENCY CARE

The attending physician is responsible for establishing a plan of emergency care for his patient. In the event that this plan fails, the administrative physician is responsible to provide for, either by himself or through a program of coverage, immediate physician service to satisfy the needs of the patient in the event of emergency. In this event, the physician responding to the emergency should provide the total medical needs required of the patient and properly record such in the progress notes and doctor's orders where necessary.

DISCHARGE

It is the responsibility of the attending physician to totally evaluate the condition of the patient at a time when it appears his needs have been totally met by the facility and indication is for him to be transferred home or to some other facility. The attending physician must make such recommendation and allow for a reasonable period of time to accomplish the discharge of the patient.

The patient should be discharged only on the written order of the attending physician and should include a discharge summary fully outlining the course of care of the patient and including a plan of continuing care following discharge.

On discharge of the patient, or within a period not to exceed one week, the attending physician should complete all sections of the medical record under his authority, including the final diagnosis, and should enter his signature to certify the accuracy of the record.

MEDICAL RECORDS

Medical records are the property of and are under the authority of the administration and must not be removed from the facility without proper and legal authority.

Medical records may be made available to certified physicians for research purposes provided that the confidence of information be provided for the patient.

REPORTABLE CONDITIONS AND COMMUNICABLE DISEASES

In accordance with state and local health requirements and authorities, information regarding those diseases and conditions determined as reportable to the proper public health unit must become available; and in all such instances it is the responsibility of the attending physician and administration to provide this reporting service.

Patients should be admitted with a questionable diagnosis of communicable disease only in order to establish more accurately the existence of, by diagnostic procedure, the communicable disease. The referring physician must certify in advance the question of such condition. Upon determination of the presence of communicable disease the attending physician must assist the administration in making necessary arrangements to protect the health of the patient by isolation pending transfer to the proper communicable disease center.

Reportable conditions such as venereal disease, gunshot wound or other eivdence of weapon assault must be recorded by the attending physician in the medical record, and, in concert with the administration, he must provide a proper report to the local health authority.

POST-MORTEM EXAMINATION

Post-mortem examinations are required in all medical-legal situations. The local medical examiner will determine the necessity of the post-mortem examination on such cases. The certifying authorities recommend a minimum of 20 per cent level of post-mortem examination for all deaths. Written consent from the nearest of kin must be obtained by the attending physician and administration before any post-mortem examination is permitted. Such examination must be performed by a certified pathologist, and a written report must be entered in the medical record.

CHAPTER FIVE

NURSING SERVICE POLICIES

PURPOSE

It is the purpose of the nursing service to assure that the total care to all patients is provided by coordination of all disciplines and skills available, each provided within a respective area of responsibility. The organization of these disciplines and skills should be directed by the nursing service in such a manner that all patients receive the most efficient and comprehensive care.

The objectives of nursing service are to assure that all the facets of patient care necessary to the health and happiness of the patients are provided. Included in these objectives are the following:

Each patient must be considered individually as to his total needs, be they physical, mental or social, with assurance that these needs are met efficiently and safely.

A current in-service teaching program should be available to all members of the staff, to the patients and to their families as an integral part of patient care.

Study and research should be supported. The results may provide better knowledge of proper care of the patients.

Those patients in need of rehabilitation should be afforded the total opportunity from skilled personnel, adequate equipment and conducive facility.

It is essential that relationships among personnel, patients, families, physicians and community be supported and maintained in the best interest of the patient.

It is the responsibility of nursing service and administration to assure that patient care is provided in accordance with the regulations of the Joint Commission on Accreditation of Hospitals and Nursing Homes and the Nursing Practice Act and in accordance with the standards of the American Nurses' Association.

DIRECTOR OF NURSES

The director of nurses is trained and experienced in areas such as nursing service administration, rehabilitation nursing and psychiatric or geriatric nursing.

The director of nurses is responsible for developing and maintaining nursing service objectives, standards of nursing practice, nursing procedure manuals and written job descriptions for each level of nursing personnel.

She (or he) recommends to the administrator the number and levels of nursing personnel to be employed and participates in their recruitment and selection and recommends termination of employment when necessary.

The director of nurses assigns and supervises all levels of nursing personnel.

She participates in planning and budgeting for nursing care.

She participates in the development and implementation of patient care policies and refers problems of patient care and policy changes to the attention of the professional policy advisory group.

She coordinates nursing services with policies and personnel of other patient care services, such as physicians, physical therapists, occupational therapists and dieticians.

She plans and conducts orientation programs for new nursing personnel and provides continuing in-service education for all nursing personnel.

She participates in the selection of perspective patients in terms of nursing services they need and nursing competencies available.

She assures that a nursing care plan is established for each patient and that this plan is reviewed and modified as necessary.

SUPERVISING NURSE

Nursing care is provided by or under the supervision of a full-time registered professional nurse currently licensed to practice in the state. Such supervising nurse is trained and experienced in areas such as nursing, administration and supervision, rehabilitation nursing and psychiatric or geriatric nursing.

The supervising nurse makes daily rounds to all nursing units, performing such functions as visiting each patient and reviewing clinical records, medication cards, patient care plans and staff assignments, and to the greatest degree possible accompanies physicians when visiting patients.

In the absence of the usual administrative authority and the director of nurses, the supervising nurse in charge of organization should be responsible for all decisions and actions in behalf of the administration.

CHARGE NURSE

There is at least one registered professional nurse or qualified licensed practical nurse who is a graduate of a state approved school of practical nursing on duty at all times and in charge of the nursing activities during each tour of duty.

The charge nurse has the ability to recognize significant changes in the condition of patients and to take necessary action.

She (or he) is responsible for the total nursing care of patients during her (his) tour of duty.

24-HOUR NURSING SERVICE

There shall be a 24-hour nursing service with a sufficient number of nursing personnel on duty at all times to meet the total needs of patients.

These nursing personnel must include registered professional nurses, licensed practical nurses, aides and orderlies.

The amount of nursing time available for patient care is exclusive of non-nursing duties.

Sufficient nursing time must be available to assure that each patient receives treatments, medications and diet as prescribed; that each patient receives proper care to prevent decubitus ulcers and is kept comfortable, clean and well groomed; that each patient is protected by the adoption of indicated safety measures from accident and injury; and that each patient is treated with kindness and respect.

Licensed practical nurses, nurses' aides and orderlies must be assigned duties consistent with their training and experience.

NURSING UNIT

A licensed registered or practical nurse must be in charge of each patient unit at all times and must be responsible for the carrying out of nursing policies and objectives. In addition, it should be the responsibility of the charge nurse to daily review patients' charts for accuracy and completeness. She must also assure that all facets of patient care are being carried out with the highest level of efficiency.

The charge nurse should report daily to the director of nurses regarding the total operation of her nursing unit, outlining specifically those unusual incidents or abnormalities that have occurred during the previous 24 hours.

RESTORATIVE NURSING CARE

There shall be an active program of restorative (rehabilitative) nursing care directed toward assisting each patient to achieve and maintain his highest level of self-care and independence. Any restorative nursing care initiated in the hospital must be continued immediately upon admission to the facility. Nursing personnel must be taught restorative nursing measures and practice them in their daily care of patients. These include

Maintaining good body alignment and proper positioning of bedfast patients.

Encouraging and assisting bedfast patients to change position at least every two hours day and night to stimulate circulation and prevent decubitus ulcers and deformities.

Making every effort to keep patients active and out of bed for reasonable periods of time, except when contraindicated by physicians' orders, and encouraging patients to achieve independence in activities of daily living by teaching self-care, transfer and ambulation activities.

Assisting patients to adjust to their disabilities, to use their prosthetic devices and to direct their interests toward self-help if necessary.

Assisting patients to carry out prescribed physical therapy exercises between visits of the physical therapist.

Utilizing consultation and instruction in restorative nursing that is available from state or local agencies.

DIETARY SUPERVISION

Nursing personnel must be aware of the dietary needs for food and fluid in patients.

Nursing personnel must make certain that patients are served diets as prescribed.

Patients needing help in eating must be assisted promptly upon receipt of meals.

Adaptive self-help devices must be provided to contribute to the patient's independence in eating.

Food and fluid intake of patients must be observed, and deviations from normal must be reported to the charge nurse.

Persistent, unresolved problems must be reported to the physician.

NURSING CARE PLAN

There must be a written nursing care plan for each patient based on the nature of his illness, treatment prescribed, long- and short-term goals and other pertinent information. The nursing care plan must be a personalized daily plan for individual patients. It should indicate what nursing care is needed, how it can best be accomplished for each patent, how the patient likes things done, what methods or approaches are most successful and what modifications are necessary to insure best results.

The nursing care plan must be available for use by all nursing personnel.

The nursing care plan must be reviewed and revised as needed.

Relevant nursing information from the nursing care plan must be included with other medical information when patients are transferred.

IN-SERVICE EDUCATIONAL PROGRAM

There must be a continuing in-service educational program in effect for all nursing personnel in addition to a thorough job orientation for new personnel.

Skilled training for non-professional nursing personnel must begin during the orientation period.

Planned in-service programs must be conducted at regular intervals for all nursing personnel.

All patient care personnel must be instructed and supervised in the care of emotionally disturbed and confused patients and must be trained to understand the social aspects of patient care.

Skilled training must include demonstration, practice and supervision of simple nursing procedures. It also must include simple restorative nursing procedures.

Orientation of new personnel must include a review of the procedures to be followed in emergencies.

Opportunities must be provided for nursing personnel to attend training courses in restorative nursing and other educational programs related to the care of long-term patients.

REHABILITATION

Immediately following the patient's admission, the physician should by examination and written statement indicate the rehabilitative potential of the patient. Such a statement should include the immediate and long-term needs and goals to be accomplished and should recommend a program to meet these goals.

The physical and occupational therapy consultants should review the recommendations of the physician, further consult with the physician regarding the program of rehabilitation and then take immediate steps to institute such a program.

The physician, during periods of his regular visit to his patient, should re-evaluate the progress of the patient, consult with the therapy consultants, review orders and certify the continuing program indicated.

BUDGET

The business office should prepare a detailed statement monthly, describing the utilization of supplies and equipment by all nursing units, including the cost of such equipment and supplies.

A regular review of the expenses of the nursing department should be held with the administration.

Regular reports should be submitted by the director of nurses to the administration recording the number of nursing hours per patient day and the average nursing hours per patient per day.

The director of nurses, the administrator and the business manager should meet at least monthly to discuss the total allocation of personnel, materials and supplies, and other financial items indicated, both for the previous month and for succeeding periods of the year.

REPORTINGS

The director of nurses should complete a daily report to be submitted to the administrator regarding the general activities of the nursing department.

The director of nurses should be ultimately responsible for insuring that all medical records are complete in accordance with the policies for maintaining clinical records and general charting procedures.

The director of nurses is responsible for necessary paperwork to be completed in accordance with nursing care policies, the scheduling of nursing personnel, all records regarding certification of hours of personnel and all necessary personnel items, including fringe benefits, vacation accrual, sick time usage, and absence from duty. The director of nurses is further responsible for recommendations on all personnel within her department regarding salary levels and increments in pay.

The director of nurses is responsible for the accuracy of bookkeeping and the recording of narcotics usage on the nursing units.

EQUIPMENT, MATERIALS AND SUPPLIES

The director of nurses is responsible for all requests to the administration for the purchase of equipment, materials and supplies.

The administration should, in turn, review regularly with the director of nurses the procedures and timing for purchases, including the selection by brand and quality of all purchases.

The director of nurses should be responsible for referring requests for all maintenance of nursing equipment and housekeeping needs on all nursing units on a regularly scheduled basis.

EMERGENCIES

The director of nurses should be responsible for the completion of all accident and incident reports on all personnel. This record should describe the reporting, course of action taken and results of all such incidents and accidents. It should be referred in the form of a daily notice to the administration.

Where an incident or accident involves a member of the personnel staff, the indicated physician should be immediately called, first aid given by the health nurse pending the arrival of the physician and correct emergency procedures followed as a result of the written order of the physician. A well-defined description should be filed in the health record of the personnel.

In the event of a patient incident or accident the indicated physician must be called, the prescribed emergency procedures followed and an adequate report recorded in the patient's medical record.

PHYSICIAN'S ORDERS

Physician's orders must be written on the doctor's order sheet at the proper intervals in a legible manner.

Telephone orders should be allowed only in cases of emergency and may be accepted only by a licensed registered or practical nurse. The ordering physician must sign the doctor's order sheet within 24 hours.

MEDICATION PROCEDURES

Licensed personnel only, under the authority of the director of nurses, shall be permitted to give medication to patients.

Errors in medications must immediately be noted and the attending physician notified. The medication error must be noted in the medical record, as well as the fact that the attending physician has been notified.

Medication must be ordered through the pharmacy under the authority of a licensed pharmacist and is delivered to the nursing unit, where the responsible nurse must check the medication for its correctness of labeling both as to medicine and patient.

The charting of medications must be done by licensed nursing personnel only.

DIETARY PROCEDURES

Diet formulas for all patients must be established under the authority of the consultant dietitian and with the approval of the attending physician.

All patients wherever possible should be encouraged to feed themselves. Assigned nursing personnel should give assistance to those patients in need of help with their meals.

The director of nurses should be responsible for obtaining reports from all nursing personnel regarding abnormalities in patient diet habits. These reports should be referred to the consultant dietitian and the attending physician.

Establishment of special diets and changes in diets must be properly recorded in the medical record, and it is the responsibility of the director of nurses to see that nursing personnel carry out these programs of diet for their patients.

TREATMENTS

All treatments to patients must be provided only upon written order of the attending physician. The order must be recorded in the patient's medical record, and evidence must appear in the order that the appropriate service, such as physical therapy, occupational therapy, laboratory or other service, has been properly notified. The procedures for carrying out such orders should be outlined in a manual for nursing procedures.

EDUCATION OF PATIENTS AND FAMILIES

A newsletter should be published periodically and should contain information of interest and importance to the patients, their families and personnel. The administration should take the opportunity in this newsletter to point out policies, to explain changes in policies, to include information that might be of value in the care of patients and the relationship of family to personnel and patients and to maintain the morale of personnel.

POSITION SUMMARY—DIRECTOR OF NURSES

The director of nurses must be responsible for the total nursing care of all patients. This care must include general nursing care, all treatments, dispensing of medicines and drugs which have been ordered by the physician and the carrying out of all doctors' orders. It is the further responsibility of the director of nurses to develop nursing objectives, standards of nursing, a nursing procedure manual and to conduct a review of these with all nursing personnel regularly. In cooperation with the administration, job descriptions for all nursing personnel must be developed. The recruitment for employment and the assignment of duties of all nursing personnel are the responsibilities of the director of nurses. In addition, the director of nurses is responsible for the planning and operation of the budget and the utilization of materials and supplies and equipment within the nursing department. The director of nurses shall be responsible for the establishment of a nursing care plan for each patient. All nursing personnel should be provided with an orientation program and a fully defined in-service educational opportunity.

QUALIFICATIONS

Duly licensed as a registered nurse in the state.

In good physical health and under the retirement age.

At least three years of experience in an administrative nursing capacity.

Demonstration of leadership ability and an ability to coordinate the activities of other nursing personnel with other personnel in other departments.

Ability to plan, develop and implement nursing policies concerning the care of patients.

Ability to coordinate the activities of the nursing department with those of all other departments.

Ability to understand and carry out policies, regulations and procedures current with the newest nursing literature and corresponding developments in the nursing profession.

Ability to apply the principles of personnel administration in the selection and assignment of nursing personnel.

Ability to adequately budget for personnel hours, materials and supplies for the department.

Ability to develop plans for coordination of nursing services with other patient care services, including physical therapy, occupational therapy, dietetics, and other ancillary services.

Ability to arrange for orientation of new personnel and provide for in-service education programs for all nursing personnel.

DUTIES

Direct all levels of nursing care.

Direct all nursing personnel.

Prepare and implement the staffing patterns and schedule hours of duty of all nursing personnel.

Supervise the duties of the charge nurses.

Chair all in-service training meetings with nursing personnel, including the recording of minutes of such meetings.

Attend regular staff meetings.

Be an active member of the professional advisory committee.

Attend all meetings and conventions necessary to the best interest of the nursing department and patients.

Require that the nursing department provide for and adhere to all nursing objectives and policies.

Consult with the attending physicians during their visits.

Provide for police reporting in the case of disorderly persons visiting nursing units.

Select and assign of all nursing personnel.

Require all nursing personnel to undergo laboratory testing and chest x-ray, with an accompanying physical examination, indicating physical capability of nursing personnel to discharge their duties.

Conduct regular examination of patients' rooms for housekeeping.

Be available to patients for counseling on nursing matters.

Conduct regular review of patients' charts.

Provide assurance that the privileges of all patients are made available to them in accordance with the policies of the administration.

Review with the consultant dietitian all special diets to assure that proper foods are being served to the patients.

Assure that all patient linen, including personal dress of patients, is of proper condition of cleanliness and appearance.

Assure that patients be allowed and encouraged to participate in religious activities of their choice.

Provide services necessary for the good grooming of all patients, including haircuts and shaves for men and hairstyles for women.

Report daily to administration on patient condition.

Report daily to administration an evaluation of nursing care given each 24 hours.

Review the employment of nursing personnel in regard to hiring of new personnel and separation of personnel from employment.

Report to administration daily the levels of personnel on duty, the number of new personnel, the number separated and all charges filed against all personnel.

Provide accident and incident reports on all personnel, patients and visitors, and provide the administration with reports of these incidents and accidents.

Report to administration all problems in connection with attending physicians.

Submit monthly census reports to administration.

Review all patients' charts in regard to supplies and services furnished, including articles broken or lost, and report circumstances surrounding any incidents concerning supplies.

POSITION SUMMARY — SUPERVISING NURSE

The supervising nurse is the immediate assistant to the director of nurses and in the absence of the director functions in her capacity. It is the responsibility of the supervising nurse to evaluate and direct the patient care. She must be constantly available to the nurses in charge of the various units and know of changes in condition of patients and the indicated action. The supervising nurse is responsible to aid in the in-service training of all nursing personnel. She is responsible for daily rounds and visiting of all patients in nursing units, for reviewing medical records, medication sheets, patient care plans and staff assignments and for cooperating with attending physicians during their visits. The supervising nurse must report daily to the director of nurses regarding all her activities.

QUALIFICATIONS

Duly registered and licensed in the state.

At least one year of experience in a supervisory capacity and some educational background in nursing administration and supervision.

Ability to lead and direct all nursing personnel in the performance of their duties.

In good physical health and under the retirement age.

Ability to coordinate the activities of the nursing units and the personnel therein.

DUTIES

Make daily rounds of all nursing units.

Visit all patients on a regular basis, preferably daily.

Implement the nursing care plans.

Review medical records, medicine sheets and physicians' orders.

Implement the plan of assignment from the director of nurses.

Record the attendance of personnel.

Accompany physicians during their visits.

POSITION SUMMARY—CHARGE NURSE

The charge nurse is responsible for carrying out the assignment of patient care on the particular nursing unit. The charge nurse must be the leader of all personnel working in the unit. The charge nurse is responsible for the dispensing of medication to all patients; for providing treatments for all patients as indicated; for receiving telephone orders from physicians; for recognizing and reporting significant changes in the condition of patients, and for taking the proper action. The charge nurse is also responsible for carrying out the nursing care plan and may be responsible for the care of assigned patients.

QUALIFICATIONS

Duly registered and licensed in the state as a registered nurse or a licensed practical nurse.

In good physical health and under the retirement age.

Ability to provide leadership and supervision to personnel within the patient unit.

Ability to recognize changes in the condition of patients and to take the actions required.

By training and experience has the ability to coordinate all the functions included in the operation of a patient unit.

DUTIES

Be responsible for the nursing care of all patients in the patient unit.

Be responsible to visit all patients each day.

Be responsible for giving medications and recording such in the patient's medical record.

Be responsible for recording of all information in medical records.

Be responsible for the narcotic cabinet and the maintaining of records on the receipt and use of narcotics.

Consult with physicians, patients and families.

Carry out nursing procedures and train and supervise the carrying out of procedures by other personnel within the unit.

POSITION SUMMARY—UNIT SECRETARY

The unit secretary, or clerk, should preferably be someone trained in clerical duties. This person may function as the secretary to the director of nurses or as the recording clerk on a patient unit. The secretary may record information in the medical record under the direction of the registered nursing personnel. The clerk may review patients' records, nursing care plan, medicine sheets and other records for their accuracy and completeness. The clerk may perform additional general clerical duties, including typing of correspondence, ordering of supplies, receiving and delivering mail and other duties of clerical nature.

QUALIFICATIONS

High school graduate with capability in typing and clerical aptitude.

In good health and under the retirement age.

Ability to receive, understand, follow out directions.

Of reasonable intelligence with acceptable personality, good manners, and tact and diplomacy.

Typing skills above average, and a reasonable knowledge of shorthand.

Knowledge of and ability to use dictating equipment.

Ability to exemplify the policies of the administration by telephone.

DUTIES

Provide for clerical aspects of admission, transfer and discharge of patients.

Answer telephone and receive and deliver messages accurately and diplomatically.

Function as receptionist at nursing unit.

Assist nursing personnel with medical record recordings, placing reports in charts, keeping statistical information correct.

Assist in receiving, storing and distributing materials for patient unit.

Assist with the distribution of flowers, mail and other items of delivery to patient unit.

Assume general responsibility for all clerical duties as delegated by the charge nurse.

POSITION SUMMARY—NURSES' AIDE OR ORDERLY

QUALIFICATIONS

Preferably high school graduate, in good health and under the retirement age.

Ability to read and write with reasonable comprehension.

Ability to perform simple mathematics.

Able to follow instructions adequately.

Willingness to learn and eagerness to achieve.

Ability to be prompt for duty and dependable.

Ability to understand policies.

Ability to give simple directions to visitors and to demonstrate and enhance the image of the administration.

PERSONAL APPEARANCE REQUIREMENTS

Must wear white, clean, well-fitting uniforms.

Must be clean and free of offensive odors.

Hair, teeth, hands, fingernails must be neat, well kept and clean.

Shoes must be white, clean and of nursing-type regulation.

Makeup must be in good taste and moderate in amount.

Jewelry should be restricted to simple rings and wrist watch.

Must be of good character and, above all, honest.

Must be able to cooperate with other personnel.

JOB REQUIREMENTS

Must have a genuine interest in nursing and a desire to attend sick people.

Should have an interest in service to mankind.

Must have patience and diplomacy in dealing with patients.

Must be alert and trained to recognize changes in condition of patients.

Must be able to withstand physical and mental strain.

Must be able to perform a variety of simple tasks, many repetitive, some involving unpleasant conditions.

Must be able to work under supervision.

Must be able to work quietly.

Must be willing to work in any nursing unit on any shift in case of emergency or when in the best interests of the nursing department and patients.

DUTIES AND RESPONSIBILITIES

Respond to patient needs under the direction of the charge nurse.

Take temperature, respiration and pulse of patients and record them in nursing chart.

Take and record weight of patients.

Provide bed bath for patients and assist in tub bath or shower for ambulatory patients.

Give adequate grooming, including hair combing, mouth washing, shampoos and assistance in cleaning teeth and dentures.

Give alcohol rubs, back massages, change bed linens, remove and discard soiled linen, service bedpans to patients, collect urine and fecal specimens.

Perform tests for diabetes with clinitest.

Record intake and output of fluids and food of patients under the direction of the charge nurse.

Maintain adequate levels of clean cool water for patients.

Clean water containers daily.

Aid in the distribution of meals to patients.

Aid in the feeding of patients.

Assist patients in walking, and transport them to other departments as necessary.

Respond to patient call system.

Distribute and arrange patients' flowers.

Distribute mail.

Clean instruments and provide for sterilization of equipment under direction of charge nurse.

Provide necessary supplies to patients, including soap, toilet tissue, towels, washcloths and the like.

Maintain linen closet.

Give aid and assistance to the charge nurse in all areas of nursing care possible whenever requested.

THE CRITICALLY ILL PATIENT

Every patient critically ill must receive the best nursing and medical care available during his period of critical illness.

When a significant change in patient condition is observed, the nursing personnel will respond by notifying the charge nurse immediately. When deemed necessary will seek assistance from her supervisor and the attending physician will be immediately notified. A full description of the change in condition will be made and the orders delivered by the physician will be carried out.

PROCEDURES

When necessary, under the direction of the physician, the nursing supervisor will notify the next of kin.

When necessary, under the direction of the physician, the nursing supervisor will notify the indicated priest, minister or rabbi.

Under the authority of the attending physician, the patient's name will be placed on the "danger list."

All emergency procedures indicated to reverse or prevent worsening of the patient's condition must be provided.

Close attention should be given to observation of the patient, particularly the vital signs, and they should be recorded regularly for changes.

Should the respiration of the patient appear to fail, the nursing supervisor will notify the attending physician immediately.

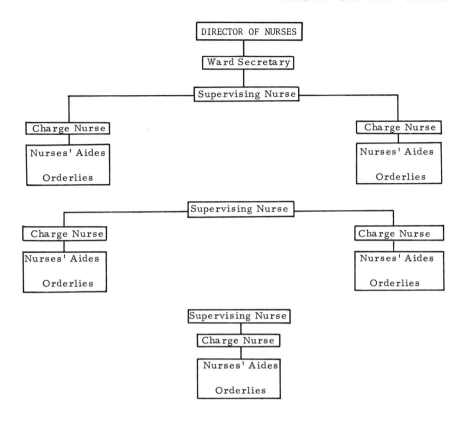

```
                    ┌─────────────────────┐
                    │ DIRECTOR OF NURSES   │
                    └─────────────────────┘
                              │
                    ┌─────────────────────┐
                    │ Ward Secretary       │
                    └─────────────────────┘
                              │
                    ┌─────────────────────┐
          ┌─────────│ Supervising Nurse    │─────────┐
          │         └─────────────────────┘          │
  ┌───────────────┐                          ┌───────────────┐
  │ Charge Nurse  │                          │ Charge Nurse  │
  ├───────────────┤                          ├───────────────┤
  │ Nurses' Aides │                          │ Nurses' Aides │
  │ Orderlies     │                          │ Orderlies     │
  └───────────────┘                          └───────────────┘

                    ┌─────────────────────┐
          ┌─────────│ Supervising Nurse    │─────────┐
          │         └─────────────────────┘          │
  ┌───────────────┐                          ┌───────────────┐
  │ Charge Nurse  │                          │ Charge Nurse  │
  ├───────────────┤                          ├───────────────┤
  │ Nurses' Aides │                          │ Nurses' Aides │
  │ Orderlies     │                          │ Orderlies     │
  └───────────────┘                          └───────────────┘

                    ┌─────────────────────┐
                    │ Supervising Nurse    │
                    ├─────────────────────┤
                    │ Charge Nurse         │
                    ├─────────────────────┤
                    │ Nurses' Aides        │
                    │ Orderlies            │
                    └─────────────────────┘
```

	NURSING CARE PLAN
GENERAL INFORMATION: M.S.W. D.Sep. RELIGION:------------------ PERSON TO NOTIFY:------------------------- RELATIONSHIP:------------------PHONE----------- ADDRESS:---------------------------------	PHYSICAL NEEDS:
SAFETY PRECAUTIONS:	
ENVIRONMENTAL ADJUSTMENTS:	INDIVIDUAL EMOTIONAL NEEDS:
PATIENT AND FAMILY TEACHING:	
NAME:	PHYSICIAN:

NURSING CARE PLAN

NH NO. RELIGION	ALLERGIES ( )	I&O ( )
DIET	AMBULATORY ( )	ORIENTED ( )
SPECIAL PROCEDURES	ASST w/DRESSING ( )	ORTHOPEDIC EQUIP:
LONG-TERM GOALS	BARBER ( )	WALKER ( ) WHEEL CHAIR ( ) TRACTION ( )
SHORT-TERM GOALS	BATH: S B T	
NURSING TEAM APPROACH	BEAUTY SHOPPE ( )	P. T. ( )
	BED ( )	POOR VISION ( )
	BED PAN ( )	RESTRAIN:
	BED RAILS ( )	NITE ( ) DAY ( )
	BLADDER IRRIG. ( )	ROM ( )
	BLOOD PRES ( )	SENSITIVE AREAS ( )
	CLINITEST ( )	SHAVE ( )
	DAILY V. S. ( )	TENDENCY TO FALL ( )
	DECUBITUS ( )	TAKE TO: O. T. ( )
	DINING ROOM ( )	CHAPEL ( ) RECREATION ( ) OUTSIDE ( )
	HAND FEED ( )	
	INCONTINENT: NITE ( ) DAY ( )	WEIGHT ( )

Name of person writing plan: _____

    PLAN WRITTEN _____   PLAN VOID _____
                (Date)   (Date)

RM #_____   NAME _____   DIAG._____

AGE _____   ADM _____   DR. _____   TEL _____

The attending physician must respond and examine the patient to determine his demise.

The attending physician, preferably, should notify the next of kin. The nursing supervisor, under the authority of the attending physician, may notify the next of kin and provide only information supplied to her by the attending physician. She must provide this to the family with utmost diplomacy in the disclosure of facts.

PATIENT CARE IN COMMUNICABLE DISEASE

In the event of an admission of a patient with a communicable disease, the object (in addition to confirmation of diagnosis) should be to provide isolation and proper treatment to patient as well as to prevent its spread to other patients.

NURSING CARE PLAN CARD
(Both front and back are shown.)

Nursing Care Plan for: Rm. No.   File No.

NEEDS	APPROACH

GOALS

Physical:	
Social:	
Psychological:	
Vocational:	
Past occupation:	
Personal interests:	

Nursing Care Card (over)

Nursing Care Plan For:

Adm. date	Birth date	Fluids
Religion	Doctor	

MEDICATIONS	Discont. Date	TREATMENT
		DIET
		Pertinent dates:
		Last Chest X-ray Doctor's visit

DIAGNOSIS:

Name   Room No.   File No.   Doctor

DAILY ASSIGNMENT CARD

DAILY ASSIGNMENT CARD

NAME AND ROOM	Bath T S B	Mouth Care	Fed	Up	Temp.	Pulse	Resp.	Turned	

PROCEDURES

Should the attending physician refer a patient for admission with a question of communicable disease, pending the confirmation of diagnosis the patient will be isolated in a single-bed room, and full isolation technique be applied. The isolation room must contain a private bath and wash sink. Proper signs must be posted on the corridor side of the door saying, "Isolation—No Visitors." All the patient's belongs shall remain in the room, preferably at bedside, to prevent spread of infection over other areas.

A rack should be placed outside the room where the physician and nursing personnel attending the patient may don isolation gowns. All personnel must wash their hands in the room at the sink prior to attending the patient and prior to leaving the patient.

All articles removed from the room must be placed in plastic bags with a significant sign stating "communicable disease," and must be disposed of sealed in the proper manner.

All bedding and linens shall be placed in isolation bags with an accompanying sign indicating contaminated linens and kept separate from other linens in their travel to the laundry. Laundering of this contaminated linen must be performed separately from the other linens.

All items of material, supplies and equipment removed from the patient's rooms must be disinfected prior to removal.

The patient must be confined to the room. Only one nursing personnel on each shift should be assigned to the patient and should be allowed to enter the room during each shift.

CARE OF THE MENTALLY DISTURBED PATIENT

It is most important to assure that any patient who becomes mentally disturbed be prevented from harming himself or others.

PROCEDURES

The nursing supervisor will make the immediate judgement as to emergency procedures regarding restraints or other measures to be taken to protect the patient from injuring himself and those around him at a time of violence due to mental disturbance.

The attending physician must be contacted immediately. Further restraining will be provided and medicines and drugs given upon the order of the physician.

An orderly should be designated to remain with the patient until the physician indicates that the patient is able to be left alone.

The transfer of a mentally disturbed patient to another facility may be indicated on the orders of the physician.

Care should be taken to provide medicines and drugs and restraints within the prescribed order to prevent the patient from harming himself or others.

PATIENT CARE POLICY FOR EMERGENCY PROCEDURES

In the event there is a medical emergency regarding a patient the following procedures should immediately be put into effect.

An immediate telephone call must be made to the attending physician or, in the event he is not available, to the administrative physician or, in his absence, to the medical exchange, asking for assistance.

In the event the patient is critically ill or there is a significant change observed in the patient's condition, the nurse in charge, following approval of the attending physician, will immediately call the patient's next of kin.

In the case of a nursing home where, in the absence of a physician, the registered nurse in charge makes a judgment as to the critical condition of the patient, she may call the rescue squad for transferral of the patient to the nearest emergency hospital.

The nurse in charge of the unit will prepare the transfer forms for the patient and will telephone the accident room of the hospital, notifying them that the patient is being transferred.

EMERGENCY NURSING PROCEDURES

The director of nurses or the supervising nurse (in charge in her absence) is responsible for the ordering of any nursing procedure considered warranted in the event of patient need. Beyond notifying the attending physician or his alternates, in his absence, and in the absence of immediate orders for the condition of the patient, the following procedures for various situations may be ordered and carried out by the nurse in charge of the unit.

Burns: Ice should be applied directly to the burn. In the event of burns more severe than first degree, particularly if there is a large area burned, either Vaseline gauze or petroleum jelly may be liberally lathered over the entire surface.

Acute diarrhea: In the event of acute diarrhea a unit dosage of Kaopectate may be given over a twenty-four hour period. Continued diarrhea warrants notification of the attending physician.

Earache: An application of warmed solution of Oralgan may be applied to the inner surface of the outer ear with a small packing of cotton loosely inserted. Should earache intensify, attending physician should be immediately notified.

Insomnia and noisiness: In the event the patient is unable to be quieted with food and soft liquids, Seconal in proper dosages may be warranted (verbal consultation with attending physician is suggested).

Lacerations: Any laceration should be immediately cleaned with a medicinal soap and water. A butterfly may be applied to halt the flow of blood. Any laceration requiring suturing should be the responsibility of the attending physician, and he should be so notified immediately.

Bruises: Ice compresses should be applied to the affected area immediately following an injury such as a fall to prevent swelling. Continued care of bruises beyond a 24-hour period should be carried out by use of warm water compresses or hot water bottle.

Fainting: Patient should be placed in a transverse Trendelenburg position in order for blood flow to be directed toward the brain. Should patient not respond within a few moments the attending physician should immediately be notified.

Coronary attacks: In the event of complaint from patient of severe chest pain, dyspnea, nausea and extreme weakness, the charge nurse should immediately notify the attending physician and prepare for the administration of oxygen pending the arrival of and orders from the physician.

Poisoning: A complete antidote chart should be available at every nurses' station with a selected checklist of medicines and drugs from the pharmacy. Following immediate medication for apparent type of poisoning the attending physician should be promptly notified.

Headache: Aspirin or Empirin compound may be given to patient for simple headache or for muscle pain or spasm. Persistent headaches warrant notification of the attending physician.

Simple indigestion: In the event of what appears to be simple indigestion, sodium bicarbonate in water may be given for relief. Continuation of symptoms may call for notification of attending physician.

Constipation—fecal impaction: In the case of simple constipation, mineral oil or milk of magnesia may be prescribed for patient. Persistent constipation resulting in fecal impaction may require low enema, using either soap solution and warm water or a prepared Fleet-type enema.

Nosebleed: Patient's head should be raised and ice pack applied to the area surrounding the nasal passages. Should bleeding not subside within one-half hour the attending physician should be notified.

REGULAR NURSING PROCEDURES

The charge nurse is responsible for the preparation and administration of all medicines and drugs to the patients in the unit.

All ambulatory patients should be encouraged to take showers or tub baths except where there are contraindications.

Care to the body of the patient is the responsibility of the nursing personnel. This responsibility includes examination of hair, nails and feet, as well as the maintenance of the entire body skin.

A regular program of temperature, pulse, respiration and blood pressure recording should be established and carried out on all patients.

Rehabilitation nursing should be applied to all patients where called for. This should include range of motion, teaching of transfer techniques and use of wheel chairs, walkers and other prosthetic devices to aid in ambulation and self care.

When authorized by the attending physician, the nursing unit personnel should make every effort to aid and assist the patient in early ambulation so that rehabilitation and discharge may be accomplished in a healthy condition.

The medical record of each patient should contain a sheet within the nursing section containing the following information:

Name of attending physician _____ M.D.
Telephone number _____
Name of administrative physician _____ M.D.
Telephone number _____
Medical Exchange telephone number _____
Name of nearest of kin _____
Address _____
Telephone number _____
Who to notify in case of emergency _____
Address _____
Telephone number _____

A suggested form for authorization to attend a patient follows:

Should I be unavailable in the event of emergency situation regarding my patient please call _____ M.D. who is my covering physician. In the event neither of us is available you are authorized to notify the administrative physician _____ M.D. or the Medical Exchange.

(Signature) _____ M.D.
Attending Physician

IN-SERVICE EDUCATION

In-service education should be provided for all levels of personnel, particularly nursing personnel, so that they may be able to better perform their services in line with the policies of the organization, and so that they may perform within the established procedures to assure that all patients receive proper nursing care.

TRAINING PROCEDURE

A selected registered nurse, preferably one with experience in in-service education, should be assigned the task of providing the orientation and immediate in-service training for all new personnel.

It is the responsibility of the director of nurses to establish a program of training that includes a description of policy and procedure for the care of patients. The following policies should be included in the training program.

A clear delineation of job description.

An organizational chart with particular attention given to the location of the various personnel within the organizational structure.

Complete orientation of personnel to the organization.

Explanation of the nursing care plan and the procedures manual.

Explanation of relationships among physician, patient and family.

Explanation of organization of business procedures.

Discussion of personal hygiene required of all personnel.

Explanation of lines of authority.

Emergency instruction, such as fire and disaster.

Description of all the services (including social services) rendered by the organization.

Evaluation of nursing personnel and their performance.

Explanation of policies of privacy of medical information.

Explanation of policies regarding use of telephone.

Explanation of functions of various administrative personnel, including administrator, director of nurses and Administrative Physician; and explanation of various committees and conferences, including utilization and nursing review.

Review of state laws pertaining to nursing.

Review of drug abuse laws.

Relationships of personnel to one another and to those above and below in authority.

Review of the rights and privileges of patients.

Review of the rights and privileges of families.

Explanation of procedures for admitting and discharging patients.

Explanation of procedures for completion of the medical record.

Explanation of procedures regarding regular and special diets.

Explanation of procedures regarding rehabilitation of patients.

Explanations of other patient care areas, such as

Recording of weight and taking of temperature, respiration, blood pressure.

Patient bathing, including tub and shower procedures.

Comfort of patients, including massages, lotion and alcohol rubs.

Care of bedclothes.
Prevention of decubitus ulcers.
Procedures in making beds for patients both in and out of bed.
Care of soiled linen, including isolation linen.
Use in care of bedpans.
Collecting specimens.
Using Clinitest and performing acid test.
Procedures for recording intake and output of fluids and foods.
Use and care of beverage service for patients.
Serving patients meals and assisting patients with eating.
Walking patients.
Answering patient call system.
Delivering messages.
Care of flowers.
Care in the cleaning and sterilizing of instruments and equipment.
Proper utilization of linen and care of linen closet.
Dressing and undressing patients.
Various activities of daily living, including self-care and self-help activities.
Aiding patients in carrying out prescribed exercises for physical therapy and occupational and diversional therapy.
Knowledge, recognition and reporting of patient's condition.
Care in the prevention of accidents and injury to patients.
Observation and reporting of eating habits of patients.
Care to prevent abuse of patient by himself, other patients or other personnel.

PROFESSIONAL RELATIONSHIP

Knowledge of the following areas:
Rehabilitative and geriatric nursing.
Physical therapy in the nursing department.
Dietetics in nursing.
Sanitation of plant and equipment.
Lines of authority.
Dental services.
Diagnostic services.
Pharmaceutical services.
Social services.
Evaluation of medical and nursing care.
Professional relationships with physicians.
Function of the administrative physician.
Laws applicable to nursing.
The art of delegating authority.
Availability and purposes of conventions, seminars and workshops.
System of reporting on meetings.

CHAPTER SIX

DIETARY SERVICES

The dietary service must be directed by a qualified individual and must be equipped to meet the daily dietary needs of patients.

DIETARY SUPERVISION

A person designated by the administrator must be responsible for the total food service of the facility. This person need not be a professional dietitian; however, in this case, regularly scheduled consultation from a professional dietitian must be obtained. A professional dietitian must meet the American Dietetic Association's qualification standards.

Other persons may be in charge of the dietary services provided they have suitable training and are graduates of baccalaureate degree programs with major studies in food and nutrition.

The person in charge of the dietary service must participate in regular conferences with the administrator and other supervisors of patient services. This person must make recommendations concerning the quantity, quality and variety of food purchased. This person is also responsible for the orientation, training and supervision of food service employees and must participate in their selection and in the formulation of pertinent personnel policy.

ADEQUACY OF DIET STAFF

There must be food service employees on duty over a period of twelve or more hours.

Food service employees must be trained to perform assigned duties and participate in selected in-service education programs.

In the event that food service employees are assigned duties outside the dietary department, these duties may not interfere with the sanitation, safety or time required for dietary work assignments.

Work assignments and duty schedules must be posted.

HYGIENE OF DIET STAFF

Food service personnel must be in good health and practice hygenic food handling techniques.

They must wear clean, washable garments and hairnets or clean caps, and hands and fingernails must be kept clean at all times.

Routine health examinations must meet local, state and federal codes for service personnel. Personnel having symptoms of communicable diseases or open, infected wounds may not be permitted to work.

ADEQUACY OF DIET

The food and nutritional needs of patients must be met in accordance with physicians' orders and must, to the extent deemed possible by the physician, meet the dietary allowances of the Food and Nutrition Board, National Research Council, based upon age, sex and amount of physical activity.

The following allowances may be used as a daily food guide for adults.

Milk—two or more cups.

Meat group—two or more servings of beef, veal, pork, lamb, poultry, fish or eggs.

Vegetable and fruit group—four or more servings of a citrus fruit or other fruit or vegetable high in vitamin C. A dark green or deep yellow vegetable (for vitamin A) at least every other day. Other vegetables and fruits, including potatoes.

Bread and cereal group—four or more servings of whole grain, enriched or restored.

—Other foods to round out meals and snacks to satisfy individual appetites and provide additional calories.

THERAPEUTIC DIETS

Therapeutic diets must be prepared and served as prescribed by the attending physician. The orders for these diets must be planned, prepared and served with supervision or consultation from a qualified dietitian.

A current diet manual must be readily available to food service personnel and supervisors of nursing service.

Persons responsible for therapeutic diets must have sufficient knowledge of food values to make appropriate substitutions when necessary.

QUALITY OF FOOD

At least three meals or their equivalent must be served daily at regular times with not more than a 14 hour span between a substantial evening meal and breakfast.

Between-meal or bedtime snacks of nourishing quality should be offered.

PLANNING OF MENUS

Menus must be planned in advance and food sufficient to meet the nutrition needs of patients must be prepared as planned for each meal.

Menu changes must provide equal nutritive value.

Menus must be written at least one week in advance and must be readily accessible in the dietary department for use by workers in purchasing, preparing and serving of food.

Menus must provide a sufficient variety of foods served in adequate amounts at each meal.

Menus must be different for the same days of each week and adjusted for seasonal changes.

Records of menus served must be filed and maintained for 30 days.

Stores of staple foods for a minimum of one week and of perishable foods for a minimum of two days must be maintained on the premises.

Records of food purchased for preparation must be on file.

PREPARATION OF FOOD

Foods must be prepared by methods that conserve nutritive value, flavor and appearance and must be attractively served at the proper temperatures in a form to meet individual needs.

A file of tested recipes, adjusted to appropriate yield, should be maintained.

Food should be cut, chopped or ground to meet individual needs.

If a patient refuses the food served, substitutes must be offered.

Effective equipment must be provided and procedures established to maintain food at proper temperature during serving.

Table service must be provided for all who can and will eat at a table, including wheelchair patients.

Trays must be provided for bedfast patients and must rest on firm supports such as over-bed tables.

Sturdy tray stands of proper height must be provided for patients able to leave their beds.

MAINTENANCE OF SANITARY CONDITIONS

Sanitary conditions must be maintained in the storage, preparation and distribution of food.

Effective procedures for cleaning all equipment and work areas must be followed consistently.

Dishwashing procedures and techniques must be well developed, understood and carried out in compliance with state and local health codes.

Written reports of inspections by state and local health authorities must remain on file in the facility, with notations made of any action taken by the facility to comply with any recommendations.

Waste, if not disposed of by mechanical means, must be kept in leakproof, nonabsorbent containers with close-fitting covers and must be disposed of daily in a manner that will prevent transmission of disease, bothersome sights or odors or the formation of a breeding place for flies or a feeding place for rodents. Containers must be thoroughly cleaned inside and out each time they are emptied.

Dry or staple food items must be stored off the floor in a well-ventilated room not subject to sewage or waste water backflow or contamination by condensation, leakage, rodents or vermin.

Hand washing facilities, including hot and cold water, soap and individual towels (preferably paper towels), must be provided in kitchen areas.

FOOD-BORNE DISEASE

Food is, of course, essential to promoting and maintaining the health and morale of facility patients. Proper precautions must be taken to prevent food from becoming a vehicle for conveying pathogenic organisms, bacterial toxins or poisonous chemicals to patients.

Meat, poultry and fish are the major causes of food-borne diseases in extended care facilities. Salmonellosis, staphylococcal food poisoning and gastroenteritis are a few of the commonly involved conditions.

FOOD-BORNE DISEASE CONTROL FACTORS

Control of food-borne diseases can be obtained by attention to the following food protection factors.

Source and wholesomeness of food. Only wholesome food from approved sources should be purchased and served.

Human factor. All food handlers must be free from any communicable disease. They must maintain a high degree of personal cleanliness and conform to hygienic practices while on duty.

Temperature-time exposure. All perishable food must be stored at temperatures that will protect against spoilage. All potentially spoilable foods shall be maintained at safe temperatures (45° F. or below, or 140° F. or above) except during necessary periods of preparation and service. All food, while being stored, prepared or served must be protected from contamination.

Sanitary design of equipment and facilities. All equipment and utensils should be so designed and of such material and workmanship as to be smooth, easily cleanable, durable, in good repair, easily accessible for cleaning, nontoxic, corrosion-resistant and relatively non-absorbent.

Cleaning and sanitization. All eating and drinking utensils must be thoroughly cleaned and sanitized after each use.

CHARACTERISTICS OF FOOD SERVICE

Need for adequate nutrition. Careful selection of foods must be made to insure that sufficient protein, vitamins and minerals are included to meet the needs of the patients. Adequate diets are necessary to increase resistance to infections. Foods must be served in an attractive manner and at suitable temperatures in order to influence the patients to eat a sufficient amount to maintain health. Patients must be allowed adequate time to consume meals without hurry.

Morale and social needs.   Food service must meet social needs as well as nutritional needs. The kitchen is the heart of the facility. Quality foods prepared in a clean environment and properly served are of utmost importance to the morale of the patients.

Tray and bedside service.   Special consideration must be given to the equipment needed, the layout of the equipment and the techniques that are required for bedside service.

Facility and equipment limitations.   Equipment designed for institutional operations is essential if efficiency and adequacy are to be expected. Light-duty, home-type equipment, although in some cases able to do the job, is not desirable. Well planned and adequately equipped facilities are essential to good management.

Supervision.   Design and management must be coupled for successful food service operation. Of the two, management is more important. Poor management will allow any well designed and properly equipped establishment to fail to reach the designed potential.

Proximity to sources of contamination.   Because of the very nature of the facility, sources of pathogenic organisms are located relatively close to food preparation areas. Alternating duties of employees between food preparation, laundering and patient care is often inefficient from the standpoint of managerial efficiency and is sometimes harmful from the standpoint of hygiene. Cleaning equipment, such as mops and sponges, and food preparation equipment, such as pots and utensils, can introduce contamination into the kitchen environment if they are used in patient areas for purposes not related to food preparation.

DISEASE CONTROL ASPECTS OF FOOD SERVICE OPERATIONS

The operational flow of the kitchen is of sanitary significance. All of the following activities are important in this regard:

Menu planning
Purchasing
Receiving
Storing
Pre-preparing
Final preparing or cooking
Holding
Serving
Cleaning and sanitary maintenance

Menu Planning

Beside the basic nutritional factors of skillful menu planning, there are some important aspects in regard to the prevention of food-borne diseases.

Leftovers.   Leftover food is found to be responsible for 95 per cent of all staphylococcal food poisoning in patients. Leftovers can be kept to a minimum by the use of tested recipes and strict attention to appropriate yield. Portion-control techniques can go a long way toward eliminating the necessity of storing large quantities of potentially hazardous leftover foods.

Menus should be flexible enough that leftovers can be incorporated into future meals. Proper storage and the flexibility of menus to use leftover foods in immediately subsequent meals will minimize the chances of growth of contaminating organisms.

Equipment and facilities. Certain items are impractical to serve if the facilities available cannot properly handle these foods. For example, cream pies should never be prepared if there is insufficient refrigerator space in which to store them during the interval between completion of baking and serving. Care should be exercised not to exceed the facility capability or capacity.

Overall menu management can be the basis for determining what equipment will be needed and how food preparation areas should be laid out. Advance menu consideration may also have a bearing on the general building design.

Purchasing

Among the numerous factors which influence purchasing are the following:
   The menus that are planned.
   Standards of quality.
   Inventory.
   Market prices.
   Season: present and future availability of foods.
   Number of employees and their skills.
   Labor costs in relation to the purchase of fresh or raw foods versus frozen
      or fabricated foods.
   Capacity and capabilities of storage facilities.
   Frequency of purchases and deliveries.
   Quantity requirements imposed by normal consumption.
Some foods, because of their nature, warrant close scrutiny of their source:

Milk and milk products. These foods should be pasteurized and must meet the standards of quality established by appropriate state and local laws.

Canned foods. The only reliable sources of canned foods are those plants in which the environment, methods of preparation and retorting practices are subject to official surveillance. Home-canned foods must be avoided.

Shellfish. All shellfish must be obtained from sources that appear on the current Public Health Service list of certified shellfish shippers or sources which are state-approved.

Poultry. Fowl are frequently infected with salmonella organisms. Poultry and poultry products, then, should come only from officially inspected sources.

Meat and meat products. These foods should be obtained only from sources which are officially inspected for wholesomeness and from plants checked for sanitation under a federal, state or local regulatory program.

Ice. Water used in the manufacture of ice must be obtained from a source that is approved by the health department. Sanitation must be practiced in the manufacture of ice. Ice makers must be located and properly installed to insure protection from sources of contamination.

Equipment

As previously stated, all equipment and utensils should be so designed and of such material and workmanship as to be smooth, easily cleanable and durable. Equipment must be in good repair, and food-contact surfaces should, in addition, be easily accessible for cleaning, non-toxic, corrosion-resistant and relatively non-absorbent.

Receiving

Receiving operations are extremely important in assuring wholesome foods, free from spoilage and infestation. Useful techniques of receiving are

Checking for evidence (such as meat inspection stamps) that foods delivered comply with specifications and quality standards.

Verifying quantities delivered.

Inspecting the delivered food for signs of insect infestation. Insect deterrents, rodent exterminators and routine residual spraying of receiving areas will aid in control.

Inspecting food for signs of spoilage, such as swollen cans, slime on meat or poultry, off color or odor, rotten or decomposed fruits and vegetables and thawed frozen foods.

Storing

The importance of storing food properly cannot be overemphasized. Pathogenic microorganisms may grow in certain foods unless these foods are properly refrigerated from the time of receipt to the time of final preparation. Control of food-borne disease, therefore, hinges on keeping potentially hazardous foods at temperatures that prevent the growth of pathogens.

Chilled storage

Potentially hazardous foods should be kept at temperatures of 45° F. or below. For extended periods of time, storage temperatures should be 42° F. or below.

Container design and construction also plays a role in chilling food. Chilling food in flat pans is conducive to rapid lowering of internal temperatures. Prompt cooling of cooked leftover foods is essential in food-borne disease control. Foods should be refrigerated while hot. Never allow foods to cool to room temperature before placing in a refrigerator. Rapid cooling in shallow containers is necessary for proper air circulation within chilling units. Shelves should not be covered with paper.

Solid foods are cooled by conduction, which is slower than cooling by convection. Sandwiches, potato salads, poultry dressings, breads, puddings, croquettes, and meat loaves, all potentially hazardous foods, cool slowly.

Frozen Storage

Freezer space must be used for storing raw foods, cooked foods prepared in advance, leftover foods or prepackaged frozen foods.

Freezing and frozen storage reduces the microbial population in foods. Temperatures of 0° F. or below should be used for frozen storage of all foodstuffs. It is essential that air space between the product and the floor and walls of the freezer be maintained. Cleanliness and sanitation in processing of frozen foods are imperative, since freezing does not sterilize food.

Cooling, defrosting and refreezing may allow renewed growth of pathogens. The danger of refreezing lies in the time the food remains at a temperature suitable for bacterial growth and not in the act of refreezing, although the structure and nutritive value are adversely affected. Rapid cooling is less likely to result in spoilage since the food remains within the dangerous temperature ranges for a shorter time.

Dry storage

Dry storage areas designed for storage of food should be used only for this purpose. Pesticides should never be stored in food storage areas. Stock rotation, orderly storage and regular inspection will supplement other insect and rodent control practices. The area must be cool, dry, well ventilated, clean, orderly and well managed.

Pre-preparing

The pre-preparation of foods must be handled in a sanitary manner. Fruits and vegetables should be thoroughly washed to remove residues of chemical sprays, deposits of soil, insects and pathogenic organisms that might be on the surface.

Cooking and Post-Cooking Preparation

Nutritious, safe and appealing food plays an important role in maintaining or restoring patients' health and in keeping morale high.

All foods (particularly potentially hazardous foods) which undergo post-cooking preparation or are served without cooking after final handling, such as potato salad or chicken salad, should be prepared with a minimum of manual contact. Such dishes are safest when prepared from chilled ingredients and served immediately or rechilled between final preparation and serving.

Thermal Destruction. Heat destroys microorganisms when applied at high enough temperatures over a sufficient period of time. Thickness, weight and consistency of food are determining factors in evaluating cooking temperatures and times. For example, pork and pork products should be heated to an internal temperature of at least 150° F. for the control of trichinosis. Also, poultry and stuffing should be heated to a minimum of 165° F. throughout, with no interruption of the initial cooking process. Dressing should be cooked separately, not inside the fowl.

Holding

Even well prepared foods of good quality can lose food value and much of their flavor and visual appeal in a prolonged holding process. A minimum time lapse between preparation and service can be achieved by careful planning, efficient methods and adequate facilities.

Potentially hazardous foods which are to be served cold should be held at temperatures of 45° F. or below from the time of preparation until serving.

From a bacteriological standpoint, hot food storage and transportation facilities should maintain temperatures of at least 140° F. to either kill or prevent multiplication of existing organisms. Some practices to avoid include the following:

> Leaving food on steam tables, warming ovens or carts with temperatures below 140° F. for long periods, particularly after serving.
>
> Either cooking on steam tables or mixing cold foods with hot foods.
>
> Heating foods on steam tables rather than heating them on proper equipment.

Serving

The quality and attractiveness of food is of major importance to patients. They are well aware of the manner in which food is served and are influenced in their eating habits by these factors. Extreme care should be taken to prevent hands or clothing from coming into contact with either the food or surfaces of utensils which will later contact food. Training and supervision of responsible employees is essential to this goal.

TYPES OF TRAY ASSEMBLY AND DISTRIBUTION.

Centralized tray service.

> Prepared food is dished up and trays are assembled at a central station or assembly line in kitchen. Soiled dishes are returned to a central dishwashing area.

Decentralized tray service.

> Foods are prepared in central kitchen and sent in bulk in heated food carts to serving pantries on the floor. Dishes are stored in the pantries and trays are assembled there. Dishwashing may be done in either the serving pantry or central kitchen area.

Centralized bulk tray service.

> Trays are set up with utensils in room-temperature items and sent to assembly area in food carts, and hot foods are transported in bulk by heated food carts. Whole foods are also transported in bulk. The trays are finally assembled at the point of service.

DINING ROOM SERVICE.   Tray service where patients can eat in groups is desirable for pleasant associations long identified with group eating. Standards require that combined recreation and dining room areas should be 25 square feet per bed for 75 per cent of the total number of beds.

ICE DISPENSING.   Ice should be handled in a sanitary manner. If it is not automatically bagged it should be dispensed from the storage units with tongs or scoops and placed in pitchers or single-use paper bags. Hands should not touch ice at any time.

Cleaning and Sanitary Maintenance

Cleanliness is of the greatest importance in all food service operations. Properly cleaned and sanitized dishes do not transmit illness. The regular effective cleaning of equipment and utensils and work surfaces minimizes the chance of food residues accumulating to support the development of microorganisms.

In addition, the life span and efficiency of equipment can be improved by careful regular cleaning.

Dishwashing procedures

Kitchen aides will be assigned to the various dining rooms, not to exceed one aide per floor.

The aide will carry a pan containing a silverware solution and place the silverware in this pan. There will be a paper bag taped to the cart for paper trash, and the cart will carry a large pan for garbage and a large pan for dishes. The aides will scrape the dishes and silverware and return to the kitchen.

Utensils must be scraped or flushed thoroughly clean in a suitable detergent solution. Then they must be rinsed free of wash water and detergent and sanitized by immersion in 170° F. water for 30 seconds, or for one minute in a solution of at least 50 parts per million chlorine at not less than 75° F., or in any other chemical sanitizing solution which has been demonstrated to be equivalent in bactericidal effectiveness, which is non-toxic and for which a suitable field test is available. A three-component sink is required for this operation.

In the kitchen, the dishwasher will take the dirty dishes to the dishwashing area and will do any additional scraping required. At this time, he will also destroy any dishes that are cracked or chipped. Then he will place the dishes, according to size and shape, in the racks. Glasses will be placed, lips down, in the racks. Silverware will be kept in solution for one-half hour.

Then the dishes and silverware will be placed into the rinse sink and rinsed with hot water.

Dishwashing machines which meet the criteria set forth in the National Sanitation Foundation standards should be considered acceptable.

Prior to loading the machine with the rinsed dishes, the operator will run the dishwasher through the complete cycle. After it has been determined that the machine is operating properly and loading the machine with the rinsed dishes, the soap dispenser will be filled and the operator will commence the cycle.

The operator will observe the temperature reading and if it does not reach 140° F on the washing cycle, he will dispense with the operation. He will report to the chef, who will see that corrective action is taken immediately.

After the washing cycle is completed, the rinse button on the machine will be pushed and the operator will again observe the gauge to be certain that the temperature reaches 180° F. In the event this temperature is not reached, the operator will follow the procedure outlined in the preceding paragraph.

The machine, after the rinse cycle is completed, is drained and cleaned.

PERSONAL SERVICE ITEMS. Carafes must be of wide-mouth construction to facilitate cleaning, inspection and filling. Personal service articles such as pitchers, carafes and glasses must be collected daily, washed and sanitized in suitable facilities. Paper cups and straws can minimize the dishwashing load. Water storage vessels should be completely emptied prior to refilling from the tap.

EVALUATING CLEANLINESS. A powder of 15 per cent phenosafranin and 85 per cent talc (by weight) is sprinkled over a surface to be tested. Water is then flushed over the surface. The residual film will be red if the surface is clean.

SANITARY MAINTENANCE SCHEDULING. Supervision by the administrator and food service manager is the key to effective routine cleaning. The best solution to the problem of maintenance is the establishment of job descriptions and organization of sanitary maintenance schedules for each worker. Cleaning procedures must be included in the schedule and must be recorded on file cards regularly available to the supervisor and employee.

Five sanitation activities useful in improving food service operations

Temperature evaluations. Temperatures employed in the preparation and storage of potentially hazardous foods must be critically evaluated. Internal food temperatures should be checked with long-stemmed bayonet dial type thermometers.

Food sampling. Sampling and laboratory examination of potentially hazardous foods are important to safe operational procedures.

Sources of food. Investigation of sources of potentially hazardous food such as milk, shellfish, meat, poultry and custard-filled products should be made on a regular basis.

Management training. The training of dietary supervisors in proper sanitation techniques and the principles of food-borne disease control is an effective management training tool.

Human factors. Preventing the ill from working and encouraging good personal hygiene for habitually good operational procedures is necessary in any institution.

CONSULTANT DIETITIAN — POSITION SUMMARY

Accreditation requires that a consultant dietitian give regular consultation both to the administration and the dietary department of the organization. This consultation should include establishment under the authority of the administrative physician and the administrator of a complete system of regular and special diets. The consultant dietitian should also be available to visit those patients requiring her services in regard to their eating habits or need of particular diet.

QUALIFICATIONS

A graduate dietitian with membership in the American Dietetic Association and with certification.

Training at the baccalaureate level in the field of food and nutrition.

Experience in the field of institutional patient care.

DUTIES

Be responsible for establishing the dietary program and the dietary formulary.

Be responsible for formulating special diets and recording them.

Be responsible for modifications of the patients' menus insofar as patient preference and palatability are concerned.

Check diets and make necessary changes at the time of regular visit to patients.

Record pertinent notes in the medical record regarding the diets of patients.

Consult with the administration, director of nurses and chef regarding food problems.

Consult with the administrative physician and any attending physician whose patient has a reason for dietary consultation.

CHIEF CHEF—POSITION SUMMARY

The chef should be responsible for consultation regularly with the consultant dietitian in regard to the establishment of diets for all patients and methods of preparation of foods to assure their quality for nourishment, attractiveness and presentation to patients. The chef is further responsible for the entire kitchen area as to physical plant, equipment, materials and supplies and for the management of all kitchen personnel.

QUALIFICATIONS

In good health and under the retirement age.

Physical capacity to transport and prepare raw foods for cooking.

Preferably one year of cooking school and several years' experience in a sizable medical institution.

A thorough knowledge of cooking for large groups of people, including regular diets and a knowledge of the meaning of special diets and their applications.

Capacity to administer personnel within the kitchen unit.

Capacity to relate to other department heads.

DUTIES

Supervise the cooking of all meals.

Supervise the selection and purchase of all foods for quality and reasonableness of cost.

Engage in supervisor services of the dietary employees in the kitchen.

Consult with consultant dietitian in the description and planning of menus.

Maintain a recipe file.

Visit patients with consultant dietitian for particular dietary problems, particularly in cooking.

Supervise the sanitation of the kitchen and food storage areas.

Conduct in-service training program for kitchen personnel.

Cooperate with administration in budgeting for food, equipment and supplies.

Review therapeutic diets with consultant dietitian.

Supervise employees for sanitation and health cards.

Attend food service seminars and workshops.

COOK — POSITION SUMMARY

Under the authority of the chef, the cook prepares all raw foods and cooks according to the procedures outlined by the chief cook and the consultant dietitian. The cook should function as the chief assistant to the chef in regard not only to the preparation and delivery of food to patients but also to the supervision of kitchen personnel and the sanitation of the kitchen area, including the physical plant, equipment and storage areas.

QUALIFICATIONS

One year's training in a cook's school.

Preferably two or more years of experience in a large medical institution where large quantities of food were prepared for large numbers of personnel.

DUTIES

Perform the actual cooking of all foods and assure that they are the same as to quality and quantity of preparation.

Be responsible for the cleaning of all areas of the kitchen, including stoves, ovens, steam jackets, work tables, sinks, serving and conveyor lines, refrigerators and freezers.

Be responsible for the storage of all raw foods in their proper storage area, including those that require refrigeration and freezing.

Assist the chef in all areas of food preparation, menu planning and delivery of food to patients.

FOOD SERVICE WORKER — POSITION SUMMARY

The food service worker performs a variety of unskilled tasks, such as sweeping and washing floors, keeping refrigerators and storerooms clean and in neat order and cleaning ranges, kettles, carts, pots and pans and other food service equipment daily. The food service worker may work in the dishwashing unit or in the food service unit, or he performs food pre-preparation tasks as assigned by the cook or assists in tray service, portioning and assembling cold foods as assigned. He may also transport food carts to patient floors. The food service worker works under close supervision.

QUALIFICATIONS

Willing to perform repetitive tasks.

Initiative in maintaining kitchen in clean and orderly condition.

Ability to work with others and to perform a variety of assigned tasks under supervision.

Skill in, and ability to learn, operation of equipment and simple food preparation tasks.

Ability to read, write, speak and follow oral and written directions.

Some kitchen experience desirable. (Usually is given continuing on-the-job instruction.)

Must know how to clean various surfaces and kinds of equipment.

WORKING ENVIRONMENT. Works in clean, well-lighted, well-ventilated kitchen. Must be able to withstand heat while working around stoves and ovens, and changes in temperature when going in and out of refrigerated or Deep-freeze areas. Must be aware of the dangers of cuts and burns while working with kitchen equipment and of falls due to wet and slippery floors.

JOB RELATIONSHIPS. Food service workers are kitchen workers in quantity food service operations or are local homemakers. This is an entry job. Promotion to cook's helper, assistant cook, dishroom supervisor, counter or tray service position is possible. The food service worker is supervised by the cook, assistant cook and food service supervisor; he supervises no one. This position may be similar to those in vegetable room, salad room or dishwashing room, or to salad tray service or counter work.

DUTIES

Adequate performance of duties assigned, such as careful and sanitary handling of dishes, equipment and food. Cleanliness of assigned work area.

Physical demands: Stands, walks, bends, lifts, carries and pushes when performing assigned duties.

May be responsible for sanitation of kitchen work areas and equipment; may wash dishes or pots and pans; may assist in food preparation and service of food to patients and personnel.

Specific types of work performed are as follows:

Prepares vegetables and fruits for cooking or service.

Obtains stock from refrigerators and storerooms as directed.

Opens cans, cartons and such for cooks.

Cleans equipment, work tables, ranges, utensils, pots and pans, floor and so forth as assigned.

May also portion cold foods for tray service and assist in tray assembly.

May transport loaded tray carts to and from patient areas.

Performs related duties as assigned.

DIETARY PERSONNEL—IN-SERVICE EDUCATION

The objective of an in-service education program for dietary personnel is to provide a practical program of training to allow personnel to perform their duties of food preparation and delivery in a manner that is both efficient and economical; and, with regard to food service, in a manner that is efficient and prompt, meals that are attractive and nutritional and that best meet the needs of the patients.

AREAS OF TRAINING

The consultant dietitian, the chef and the administration should together provide in-service training for all dietary personnel in the following areas:

Food preparation.
Food handling.
Personal cleanliness.
Infections, cuts, sores.
Food poisoning.
Contamination of food.
Diabetic problems.
Food costs and food waste.
Security to kitchen.
Prohibition of unauthorized personnel from kitchen area, including nursing personnel and patients.
Technique of dishwashing.
Care of stainless steel.
Cleaning and storage of silverware.
Pot and pan washing.
Proper uniform, including hairnets, caps.
Care of mops and cleaning utensils.
Storage of equipment and supplies.
Maintenance of equipment.
Care of conveyor lines.
Care and operation of coffee machine.
Care of steam jacket, steam pots.
Cleaning exhaust filters
Cleaning exhaust hoods.
Cleaning refrigerators and freezers.
Care and cleaning of garbage cans.
Maintenance of kitchen floors and walls.
Procedures in handling tray service.
Procedures in making salads.
Procedures in preparing trays in advance, including bread, butter.
Procedures in keeping hot foods hot and cold foods cold.
Procedures in busing dishes.
Knowledge of safety procedures.
Training in relationship with other personnel.
Training in cleanliness of work.
Training in emergency procedures, including fire, disaster.
Training and knowledge of organizational chart.
Training in knowledge of job descriptions.
Training in general knowledge of the operation of dietary department, as well as general operation of the facility.

A committee comprised of the administrator, consultant dietitian, chef, and administrative physician shall review the in-service training program on a semiannual basis.

PHYSICIAN'S DIET REQUEST FORM

Patient's Name _____ Room Number _____

Physician's Name _____

Date _____

QUALITATIVE ORDER

Frequency of Feedings   *House Diets*

Three Meals _____   Normal _____

Three Meals Plus Between-

   Meal Feedings _____   Clear Liquid _____

Three Meals Plus

   Night Feeding _____   Full Liquid _____

Feedings Every Two Hours _____   Soft _____

Feedings Every Two Hours _____   Bland _____

Other _____   Mechanical _____

                                   Calorie-Restricted _____

                                   Low-Fat _____

                                   Low-Cholesterol or Fat-Controlled _____

                                   Sodium-Restricted-1000 mg. _____

                                   Tube Feeding _____

QUANTITATIVE ORDER

Check Diet Order	Diabetic Diets Calories	Carbo-hydrates	Protein	Fat	Sodium
_____	1200	125	70	50	
_____	1500	150	70	70	
_____	1800	180	80	80	
_____	2200	220	90	100	
	Restricted Calories				
_____	1000		70	20	

OTHER _____

DIETS MODIFIED FROM THE REGULAR MENU
(VARIATIONS FROM THE REGULAR MENU ARE IN PARENTHESES)

SUNDAY REGULAR MENU	SOFT OR BLAND
MORNING	
Orange Juice—½ cup	Orange Juice—½ cup
OR Grapefruit Sections—½ cup	
Cornflakes—¾ cup	Cornflakes—¾ cup
OR Farina—½ cup	
Poached Egg—1	Poached Egg—1
Crisp Bacon—2 slices	Crisp Bacon—2 slices
Toast—1 slice	Toast—1 slice
Butter or Margarine—1 pat	Butter or Margarine—1 pat
Honey—2 tsp.	Honey—2 tsp.
Coffee or Tea	Coffee or Tea (Soft Diets)
	Decaffeinated Coffee (Bland Diets)
Milk—1 cup	Milk—1 cup
Cream and Sugar—as desired	Cream and Sugar—as desired
NOON	
Bouillon—½ cup	Bouillon—½ cup (Soft Diets)
Roast Sirloin of Beef au Jus—3 oz.	Roast Sirloin of Beef—3 oz.
OR Fried Chicken—4 oz.	
Mashed Potatoes—½ cup	Mashed Potatoes—½ cup
	(Buttered Diced Carrots—½ cup)
Chef's Salad, Vinaigrette Dressing	
OR Stuffed Prune Salad	
Butterscotch Sundae	Butterscotch Sundae
OR Canned Pineapple in Syrup—½ cup	
Bread—1 slice	Bread—1 slice
Butter or Margarine—1 pat	Butter or Margarine—1 pat
Coffee or Tea	Coffee or Tea (Soft Diets)
	Milk—1 cup (Bland Diets)
Cream and Sugar—as desired	Cream and Sugar—as desired
NIGHT	
Broiled Hamburger Steak, Catsup—3 oz.	Broiled Hamburger Steak—3 oz.
OR Ham Salad, Stuffed Olives—½ cup	
Baked Potato—1 medium	Baked Potato—1 medium
Seasoned Green Beans—½ cup	(Buttered Green Beans—½ cup)
OR Buttered Diced Turnips—½ cup	
Coleslaw with Celery Seed Dressing	
OR Pear–Mint Jelly Salad, Mayonnaise	Pear–Mint Jelly Salad, Mayonnaise
Canned Fruit Cup—½ cup	
OR Banana Gelatin, Whipped Cream—½ cup	Banana Gelatin, Whipped Cream—½ cup
Bread—1 slice	Bread—1 slice
Butter or Margarine—2 pats	Butter or Margarine—2 pats
Coffee or Tea	Coffee or Tea (Soft Diets)
Milk—1 cup	Milk—1 cup
Cream and Sugar—as desired	Cream and Sugar—as desired

DIETS MODIFIED FROM THE REGULAR MENU
(Variations from the regular menu are in parentheses)

Low Fat (35 grams fat— No fat added in cooking)	1000 Calorie (No fat or sugar added in cooking)	1000 mg. Sodium (No salt, soda, baking powder or salted fat added in cooking (including baking) or other preparation. When more than 3 slices of bread are served in a day, the extra slices must be low-sodium bread. LS means low sodium. All canned vegetables should be LS.)
MORNING		
Orange Juice—½ cup	Orange Juice—½ cup	Orange Juice—½ cup (Puffed Rice—¾ cup)
Cornflakes—¾ cup	Cornflakes—¾ cup	
	OR Toast—1 slice	
Poached Egg—1	Poached Egg—1	(LS Poached Egg—1)
Toast—1 slice		Toast—1 slice
		(LS Butter or LS Margarine—1 pat)
Honey—2 tsp.		Honey—2 tsp.
Coffee or Tea	Coffee or Tea	Coffee or Tea
(Skim Milk—1 cup)	(Skim Milk—1 cup)	Milk—1 cup
Sugar—as desired		Cream—(1 tbsp. if desired)
		Sugar—as desired
NOON		
(Fat-Free Bouillon—½ cup)	(Fat-Free Bouillon—½ cup)	
Roast Sirloin of Beef—3 oz.	Roast Sirloin of Beef—3 oz.	(LS Roast Sirloin of Beef—2 oz.)
(Boiled Potato—½ cup)		(LS Mashed Potatoes—½ cup)
(Diced Carrots—½ cup)	(Diced Carrots—½ cup)	
Chef's Salad, (Low-Calorie Dressing)	Chef's Salad, (Low-Calorie Dressing)	Chef's Salad, (Special LS Dressing)
Canned Pineapple in Syrup— ½ cup	(Canned Pineapple, Art. Sweet.—½ cup)	Canned Pineapple in Syrup— ½ cup
Bread—1 slice		Bread—1 slice
(Jelly—2 tsp.)		(LS Butter or LS Margarine—1 pat)
Coffee or Tea	Coffee or Tea	Coffee or Tea
		Cream—(1 tbsp. if desired)
Sugar—as desired		Sugar—as desired
NIGHT		
Broiled Hamburger Steak—3 oz.	Broiled Hamburger Steak—3 oz.	(LS Broiled Hamburger Steak—2 oz.)
Baked Potato—1 medium		Baked Potato—1 medium
(Green Beans—½ cup)	(Green Beans—½ cup)	(LS Buttered Green Beans—½ cup)
Coleslaw with Celery Seed, (Low-Calorie Dressing)	Coleslaw with Celery Seed, (Low-Calorie Dressing)	Coleslaw, (LS Vinegar Dressing)
Canned Fruit Cup—½ cup	(Canned Fruit Cup, Art. Sweet.— ½ cup)	Canned Fruit Cup—½ cup
Bread—1 slice	Bread—1 slice	Bread—1 slice
(Jelly—2 tsp.)		(LS Butter or LS Margarine—2 pats)
Coffee or Tea	Coffee or Tea	Coffee or Tea
(Skim Milk—1 cup)	(Skim Milk—1 cup)	Milk—1 cup
Sugar—as desired		Cream—(1 tbsp. if desired)
		Sugar—as desired

DIETS MODIFIED FROM THE REGULAR MENU
(VARIATIONS FROM THE REGULAR MENU ARE IN PARENTHESES)

MONDAY

REGULAR MENU	SOFT OR BLAND
MORNING	
Orange Juice — ½ cup	Orange Juice — ½ cup
OR Half Grapefruit	
Farina — ½ cup	Farina — ½ cup
OR Dry Malt Cereal — ¾ cup	
Sausage Links — 2	(Poached Egg — 1)
Toast — 1 slice	Toast — 1 slice
Butter or Margarine — 1 pat	Butter or Margarine — 1 pat
Jelly — 2 tsp.	Jelly — 2 tsp.
Coffee or Tea	Coffee or Tea (Soft Diets)
	Decaffeinated Coffee (Bland Diets)
Milk — 1 cup	Milk — 1 cup
Cream and Sugar — as desired	Cream and Sugar — as desired
NOON	
Fresh Vegetable Soup — ½ cup	(Strained Vegetable Soup — ½ cup)
Crackers — 2	Crackers — 2
Baked Veal Steak — 2 oz.	Baked Veal Steak — 2 oz.
OR Broiled Canadian Bacon — 2 oz.	
Parsley Buttered Potato — 1 medium	Parsley Buttered Potato — 1 medium
	(Buttered Green Peas — ½ cup)
Pineapple–Marshmallow–Date Salad	
OR Celery Cabbage Salad, French Dressing	
Butterscotch Meringue Pudding — ½ cup	Butterscotch Meringue Pudding — ½ cup
OR Canned Apricot Halves in Syrup — ½ cup	
Bread — 1 slice	Bread — 1 slice
Butter or Margarine — 1 pat	Butter or Margarine — 1 pat
Coffee or Tea	Coffee or Tea (Soft Diets)
	Milk — 1 cup (Bland Diets)
Cream and Sugar — as desired	Cream and Sugar — as desired
NIGHT	
Roast Leg of Lamb — 3 oz.	Roast Leg of Lamb — 3 oz.
OR Chicken Cutlet, Cream Sauce — 4 oz.	
Whipped Potatoes — ½ cup	Whipped Potatoes — ½ cup
Buttered Asparagus Spears — ½ cup	Buttered Asparagus Spears — ½ cup
OR Buttered Succotash — ½ cup	
Carrot and Raisin Salad	
OR Pear-Toasted Coconut Salad, Mayonnaise	
Applesauce — ½ cup	Applesauce — ½ cup
OR Blueberry Cobbler	
Parker House Roll	Parker House Roll — 1
Butter or Margarine — 1 pat	Butter or Margarine — 1 pat
Coffee or Tea	Coffee or Tea (Soft Diets)
Milk — 1 cup	Milk — 1 cup
Cream and Sugar — as desired	Cream and Sugar — as desired

DIETS MODIFIED FROM THE REGULAR MENU
(VARIATIONS FROM THE REGULAR MENU ARE IN PARENTHESES)

LOW FAT (35 grams fat— No fat added in cooking)	1000 CALORIE (No fat or sugar added in cooking)	1000 MG. SODIUM (No salt, soda, baking powder or salted fat added in cooking (including baking) or other preparation. When more than 3 slices of bread are served in a day, the extra slices must be low-sodium bread. LS means low sodium. All canned vegetables should be LS.)
MORNING		
Orange Juice—½ cup	Orange Juice—½ cup	Orange Juice—½ cup
Farina—½ cup	Farina—½ cup OR Toast—1 slice	(LS Farina—½ cup)
(Poached Egg—1) Toast—1 slice	(Poached Egg—1)	(LS Poached Egg—1) Toast—1 slice (LS Butter or LS Margarine—1 pat)
Jelly—2 tsp. Coffee or Tea	Coffee or Tea	Jelly—2 tsp. Coffee or Tea
(Skim Milk—1 cup) Sugar—as desired	(Skim Milk—1 cup)	Milk—1 cup Cream—(1 tbsp. if desired) Sugar—as desired
NOON		
(Fat-Free Vegetable Soup—½ cup) Crackers—2	(Fat-Free Vegetable Soup—½ cup)	
Baked Veal Steak—2 oz.	Baked Veal Steak—3 oz.	(LS Baked Veal Steak—2 oz.)
(Parsley Potato—1 medium)		(LS Parsley Buttered Potato—1 medium)

(Green Peas—½ cup)
Celery Cabbage Salad,
    (Low-Calorie Dressing)
	(Green Peas—½ cup)
	Celery Cabbage Salad,
	    (Low Calorie Dressing)
		(LS Buttered Green Peas—½ cup)
		Celery Cabbage Salad,
		    (Special LS Dressing)

Canned Apricot Halves in
    Syrup—½ cup
Bread—1 slice
(Jelly—2 tsp.)
Coffee or Tea
	(Canned Apricot Halves, Art.
	    Sweet.—4 halves)
	
	Coffee or Tea
		Canned Apricot Halves in Syrup—
		    ½ cup
		Bread—1 slice
		(LS Butter or LS Margarine—1 pat)
		Coffee or Tea
		Cream—(1 tbsp. if desired)

Sugar—as desired		Sugar—as desired
NIGHT		
Roast Leg of Lamb—3 oz.	Roast Leg of Lamb—3 oz.	(LS Roast Leg of Lamb—2 oz.) (LS Whipped Potatoes—½ cup)
(Asparagus Spears—½ cup) (Succotash—½ cup) (Carrot Sticks—5 to 8)	(Asparagus Spears—½ cup)	(LS Buttered Asparagus Spears— 1 cup)
		Pear-Toasted Coconut Salad, (Special LS Dressing)
Applesauce—½ cup Parker House Roll—1 (Jelly—2 tsp.) Coffee or Tea (Skim Milk—1 cup) Sugar—as desired	(Applesauce, Art. Sweet.—½ cup) Parker House Roll—1 Coffee or Tea (Skim Milk—1 cup)	Applesauce—½ cup Parker House Roll—1 (LS Butter or LS Margarine—1 pat) Coffee or Tea Milk—1 cup Cream—(1 tbsp. if desired) Sugar—as desired

DIETS MODIFIED FROM THE REGULAR MENU
(Variations from the regular menu are in parentheses)

Tuesday

Regular Menu	Soft or Bland
MORNING	
Half Grapefruit	
OR Orange Juice—1 cup	Orange Juice—1 cup
Oatmeal—1 cup	
OR Corn Flakes—¾ cup	Corn Flakes—¾ cup
Soft Cooked Egg—1	Soft Cooked Egg—1
Crisp Bacon—2 slices	Crisp Bacon—2 slices
Cinnamon Roll—1	(Toast—1 slice)
Butter or Margarine—1 pat	Butter or Margarine—1 pat
Coffee or Tea	Coffee or Tea (Soft Diets)
	Decaffeinated Coffee (Bland Diets)
Milk—1 cup	Milk—1 cup
Cream and Sugar—as desired	Cream and Sugar—as desired
NOON	
Beef Stew with Vegetables—5 oz.	(Braised Beef Cubes, Lean—3 oz.)
OR Salad Plate with Cottage Cheese, Cold Cuts, and Sliced Tomato	
Baked Potato—1 medium	Baked Potato—1 medium
	(Buttered Sliced Carrots—1 cup)
Peach Cup Salad, Mayonnaise	Peach Cup Salad, Mayonnaise
OR Head Lettuce Salad, French Dressing	
Pineapple Tidbits—½ cup	
OR Chocolate Brownie (no nuts)—1	Chocolate Brownie (no nuts)—1
Roll—1	Roll—1
Butter or Margarine—2 pats	Butter or Margarine—2 pats
Coffee or Tea	Coffee or Tea (Soft Diets)
	Milk—1 cup (Bland Diets)
Cream and Sugar—as desired	Cream and Sugar—as desired
NIGHT	
Cream of Pea Soup—½ cup	Cream of Pea Soup—½ cup
Crackers—2	Crackers—2
Salisbury Steak, Catsup—3 oz.	
OR Broiled Calves' Liver, Onion Gravy—3 oz.	Broiled Calves' Liver—3 oz.
Buttered Rice—½ cup	Buttered Rice—½ cup
Buttered Sliced Beets—½ cup	Buttered Sliced Beets—½ cup
OR Buttered Cauliflower—½ cup	
Waldorf Salad	
OR Chef's Salad, French Dressing	
Cherry Shortcake, Whipped Cream	
OR Bartlett Pear Half in Syrup	Bartlett Pear Half in Syrup
Bread—1 slice	Bread—1 slice
Butter or Margarine—1 pat	Butter or Margarine—1 pat
Coffee or Tea	Coffee or Tea (Soft Diets)
Milk—1 cup	Milk—1 cup
Cream and Sugar—as desired	Cream and Sugar—as desired

DIETS MODIFIED FROM THE REGULAR MENU
(VARIATIONS FROM THE REGULAR MENU ARE IN PARENTHESES)

LOW FAT (35 grams fat— No fat added in cooking)	1000 CALORIE (No fat or sugar added in cooking)	1000 MG. SODIUM (No salt, soda, baking powder or salted fat added in cooking (including baking) or other preparation. When more than 3 slices of bread are served in a day, the extra slices must be low-sodium bread. LS means low sodium. All canned vegetables should be LS.)
MORNING		
Half Grapefruit	Half Grapefruit	Half Grapefruit
Corn Flakes—¾ cup	Corn Flakes—¾ cup	(Shredded Wheat—1 biscuit)
	OR (Toast—1 slice)	
Soft Cooked Egg—1	Soft Cooked Egg—1	Soft Cooked Egg—1
(Toast—1 slice)		(Toast—1 slice)
(Preserves—2 tsp.)		(LS Butter or LS Margarine—1 pat)
Coffee or Tea	Coffee or Tea	Coffee or Tea
(Skim Milk—1 cup)	(Skim Milk—1 cup)	Milk—1 cup
Sugar—as desired		Cream—(1 tbsp. if desired)
		Sugar—as desired
NOON		
(Braised Beef Cubes, Lean—3 oz.	(Salad Plate with Cottage Cheese (½ cup), Cold Cuts (1 slice), Sliced Tomato, Low-Calorie Dressing)	(LS Braised Beef Cubes—2 oz.)
Baked Potato—1 medium		Baked Potato—1 medium
(Broccoli—½ cup)	(Broccoli—½ cup)	(LS Buttered Broccoli—½ cup)
Head Lettuce Salad		Head Lettuce Salad
(Low-Calorie Dressing)		(Special LS Dressing)
Pineapple Tidbits—½ cup	(Pineapple Tidbits, Art. Sweet.—½ cup)	Pineapple Tidbits—½ cup
Roll—1		Roll—1
(Honey—2 tsp.)		(LS Butter or LS Margarine—1 pat)
Coffee or Tea	Coffee or Tea	Coffee or Tea
		Cream—(1 tbsp. if desired)
Sugar—as desired		Sugar—as desired
NIGHT		
Broiled Calves' Liver—3 oz.	Broiled Calves' Liver—3 oz.	(LS Salisbury Steak—2 oz.)
(Rice—½ cup)	(Sliced Beets—½ cup)	(LS Buttered Cauliflower—½ cup)
		(LS Waldorf Salad with Lemon Juice)
Chef's Salad, (Low-Calorie Dressing)	Chef's Salad, (Low-Calorie Dressing)	
Bartlett Pear Half Half in Syrup	(Bartlett Pear Halves, Art. Sweet.—2	Bartlett Pear Half in Syrup
Bread—1 slice	Bread—1 slice	Bread—1 slice
(Jelly—2 tsp.)		(LS Butter or LS Margarine—1 pat)
Coffee or Tea	Coffee or Tea	Coffee or Tea
(Skim Milk—1 cup)	(Skim Milk—1 cup)	Milk—1 cup
Sugar—as desired		Cream—(1 tbsp. if desired)
		Sugar—as desired

DIETS MODIFIED FROM THE REGULAR MENU
(VARIATIONS FROM THE REGULAR MENU ARE IN PARENTHESES)

WEDNESDAY	
REGULAR MENU	**SOFT OR BLAND**

MORNING	
Tomato Juice—½ cup	Tomato Juice—½ cup
OR Orange Halves—2	
Cooked Malt Cereal—½ cup	Cooked Malt Cereal—½ cup
OR Puffed Rice—1 cup	
Grilled Ham Slice—1 oz.	(Poached Egg—1)
Toast—1 slice	Toast—1 slice
Butter or Margarine—1 pat	Butter or Margarine—1 pat
Coffee or Tea	Coffee or Tea (Soft Diets)
	Decaffeinated Coffee (Bland Diets)
Milk—1 cup	Milk—1 cup
Cream and Sugar—as desired	Cream and Sugar—as desired
NOON	
Cranberry Juice Cocktail—½ cup	Cranberry Juice Cocktail—½ cup
	(Soft Diets)
Broiled Perch Filet, Lemon—2 oz.	Broiled Perch Filet, Lemon—2 oz.
OR Roast Loin of Pork—2 oz.	
Steamed Potato in Jacket—1 medium	Steamed Potato in Jacket—1 medium
	(Buttered Chopped Spinach—½ cup)
Citrus Fruit Salad	
OR Assorted Relishes	
Lime Sherbet—½ cup	Lime Sherbet—½ cup
OR Spice Cake, Maple Frosting	
Bread, Whole Wheat—1 slice	(Bread, White—1 slice)
Butter or Margarine—2 pats	Butter or Margarine—2 pats
Coffee or Tea	Coffee or Tea (Soft Diets)
	Milk—1 cup (Bland Diets)
Cream and Sugar—as desired	Cream and Sugar—as desired
NIGHT	
Roast Chicken—3 oz.	Roast Chicken—3 oz.
OR Veal Fricassee—4 oz.	
Buttered Noodles—½ cup	Buttered Noodles—½ cup
OR Buttered Rice—½ cup	
Scalloped Tomatoes—½ cup	
OR Buttered Green Peas—½ cup	Buttered Green Peas—½ cup
Melon-ball Salad	(Pear Half with Cottage Cheese—¼ cup)
OR Cottage Cheese with Chives	
Italian Prune Plums—½ cup	
OR Floating Island	Floating Island
Biscuit—1	(Bread—1 slice)
Butter or Margarine—1 pat	Butter or Margarine—1 pat)
Coffee or Tea	Coffee or Tea (Soft Diets)
Milk—1 cup	Milk—1 cup
Cream and Sugar—as desired	Cream and Sugar—as desired

DIETS MODIFIED FROM THE REGULAR MENU
(VARIATIONS FROM THE REGULAR MENU ARE IN PARENTHESES)

LOW FAT (35 grams fat— No fat added in cooking)	1000 CALORIE (No fat or sugar added in cooking)	1000 MG. SODIUM (No salt, soda, baking powder or salted fat added in cooking (including baking) or other preparation. When more than 3 slices of bread are served in a day, extra slices must be low-sodium bread. LS means low sodium. All canned vegetables should be LS.)
MORNING		
Tomato Juice—½ cup		
	Orange Halves—2	Orange Halves—2
Cooked Malt Cereal—½ cup		
		Puffed Rice—1 cup
(Poached Egg—1)	Grilled Ham Slice—1 oz.	(LS Poached Egg—1)
Toast—1 slice	Toast—1 slice	Toast—1 slice
(Jelly—2 tsp.)		(LS Butter or LS Margarine—1 pat)
Coffee or Tea	Coffee or Tea	Coffee or Tea
(Skim Milk—1 cup)	(Skim Milk—1 cup)	Milk—1 cup
Sugar—as desired		Cream—(1 tbsp. if desired)
		Sugar—as desired
NOON		
Cranberry Juice Cocktail—½ cup	(Cranberry Juice Cocktail, Art. Sweet.—½ cup)	Cranberry Juice Cocktail—½ cup
Broiled Perch Filet, Lemon—2 oz.	Broiled Perch Filet, Lemon—3 oz.	(LS Broiled Fresh Whitefish Filet, Lemon—2 oz.)
Steamed Potato in Jacket— 1 medium		Steamed Potato in Jacket— 1 medium
	(Chopped Spinach—½ cup)	
Citrus Fruit Salad, (Low- Calorie Dressing)	Relishes (radishes, green onions, green pepper strips)	Relishes (radishes, green onions, green pepper strips)
Lime Sherbet—½ cup	(Raw Apple—1 small)	(Raw Apple—1)
Bread, Whole Wheat—1 slice		Bread, Whole Wheat—1 slice
(Jelly—2 tsp.)		(LS Butter or LS Margarine—1 pat)
Coffee or Tea	Coffee or Tea	Coffee or Tea
		Cream—(1 tbsp. if desired)
		Sugar—as desired
NIGHT		
Roast Chicken—3 oz.	Roast Chicken—3 oz.	(LS Roast Chicken—2 oz.)
(Noodles—½ cup)		(LS Buttered Noodles—½ cup)
	(Chilled Canned Tomatoes— ½ cup)	(LS Scalloped Tomatoes—½ cup)
(Green Peas—½ cup)	(Green Peas—½ cup)	
Melon-ball Salad, (Low- Calorie Dressing)	(Leaf Lettuce, Low-Calorie Dressing)	Melon-ball Salad, (Special LS Dressing)
Italian Prune Plums—½ cup	(Italian Prune Plums, Art. Sweet.—2)	Italian Prune Plums—½ cup
Biscuit—1	Biscuit—1	(Bread—1 slice)
(Jelly—2 tsp.)		(LS Butter or LS Margarine—1 pat)
Coffee or Tea	Coffee or Tea	Coffee or Tea
(Skim Milk—1 cup)	(Skim Milk—1 cup)	Milk—1 cup
Sugar—as desired		Cream—(1 tbsp. if desired)
		Sugar—as desired

DIETS MODIFIED FROM THE REGULAR MENU
(VARIATIONS FROM THE REGULAR MENU ARE IN PARENTHESES)

THURSDAY

REGULAR MENU	SOFT OR BLAND
MORNING	
Orange Juice—½ cup	Orange Juice—½ cup
OR Fresh Frozen Strawberries—½ cup	
Farina—½ cup	Farina—½ cup
OR Dry Oat Flakes—¾ cup	
Scrambled Egg—1	Scrambled Egg—1
Raisin Toast—1 slice	(Toast—1 slice)
Butter or Margarine—1 pat	Butter or Margarine—1 pat
Coffee or Tea	Coffee or Tea (Soft Diets)
	Decaffeinated Coffee (Bland Diets)
Milk—1 cup	Milk—1 cup
Cream and Sugar—as desired	Cream and Sugar—as desired
NOON	
Baked Meat Loaf—2 oz.	
OR Welsh Rarebit with Crisp Bacon—½ cup	Welsh Rarebit with Crisp Bacon—½ cup,
on Toast Points	on Toast Points
Oven-Browned Potato—1 medium	Oven-Browned Potato—1 medium
	(Mashed Baked Winter Squash—½ cup)
Tomato-Cucumber Salad, Olive French Dressing	
OR Fresh Fruit Salad, Mayonnaise	
Royal Anne Cherries—½ cup	Royal Anne Cherries—½ cup
Vanilla Wafers—2	Vanilla Wafers—2
OR Peach Cobbler	
Plain Muffin—1	Plain Muffin—1
Butter or Margarine—1 pat	Butter or Margarine—1 pat
Coffee or Tea	Coffee or Tea (Soft Diets)
	Milk—1 cup (Bland Diets)
Cream and Sugar—as desired	Cream and Sugar—as desired
NIGHT	
Chicken Broth with Rice—½ cup	Chicken Broth with Rice—½ cup
	(Soft Diets)
Crackers—2	Crackers—2 (Soft Diets)
Broiled Lamb Patty, Mint Jelly—3 oz.	Broiled Lamb Patty, Mint Jelly—3 oz.
OR Ham a la King on Corn Bread—4 oz.	
Mashed Potatoes—½ cup	Mashed Potatoes—½ cup
Seasoned Green Beans—½ cup	Seasoned Green Beans—½ cup
OR Seasoned Shredded Cabbage—½ cup	
Lettuce Wedge, Roquefort Dressing	
OR Molded Fruit Salad	
Half Grapefruit	
OR Butter Pecan Ice Cream—½ cup	(Vanilla) Ice Cream—½ cup
Corn Bread—1 square	
OR Bread—1 slice	Bread—1 slice
Butter or Margarine—1 pat	Butter or Margarine—1 pat
Coffee or Tea	Coffee or Tea (Soft Diets)
Milk—1 cup	Milk—1 cup
Cream and Sugar—as desired	Cream and Sugar—as desired

DIETS MODIFIED FROM THE REGULAR MENU
(Variations from the regular menu are in parentheses)

Low Fat (35 grams fat — No fat added in cooking)	1000 Calorie (No fat or sugar added in cooking)	1000 mg. Sodium (No salt, soda, baking powder or salted fat added in cooking (including baking) or other preparation. When more than 3 slices of bread are served in a day, the extra slices must be low-sodium bread. LS means low sodium. All canned vegetables should be LS.)
MORNING		
Orange Juice — ½ cup	Orange Juice — ½ cup	Orange Juice — ½ cup
Farina — ½ cup	Farina — ½ cup OR (Toast — 1 slice)	(LS Farina — ½ cup)
Scrambled Egg — 1	Scrambled Egg — 1	(LS Scrambled Egg — 1)
Raisin Toast — 1 slice		(Toast — 1 slice)
(Jelly — 2 tsp.)		(LS Butter or LS Margarine — 1 pat)
Coffee or Tea	Coffee or Tea	Coffee or Tea
(Skim Milk — 1 cup)	(Skim Milk — 1 cup)	Milk — 1 cup
Sugar — as desired		Cream — (1 tbsp. if desired)
NOON		
Baked Meat Loaf — 2 oz.	Baked Meat Loaf — 3 oz.	(LS Baked Meat Loaf — 2 oz.)
Oven-Browned Potato — 1 medium		(LS Oven-Browned Potato — 1 medium)
(Mashed Baked Winter Squash — ½ cup)	(Mashed Baked Winter Squash — ½ cup)	(LS Mashed Baked Winter Squash — ½ cup)
Tomato-Cucumber Salad, (Low-Calorie Dressing)	Tomato-Cucumber Salad, (Low-Calorie Dressing)	Tomato-Cucumber Salad, (Special LS Dressing)
Royal Anne Cherries — ½ cup	(Royal Anne Cherries, Art. Sweet. — ½ cup)	Royal Anne Cherries — ½ cup
Vanilla Wafers — 2		
Plain Muffin — 1		(Bread — 1 slice)
(Marmalade — 2 tsp.)		(LS Butter or LS Margarine — 1 pat)
Coffee or Tea	Coffee or Tea	Coffee or Tea
		Cream — (1 tbsp. if desired)
Sugar — as desired		Sugar — as desired
NIGHT		
(Fat-Free Chicken Broth with Rice — ½ cup)	(Fat-Free Chicken Broth — ½ cup)	
Crackers — 2		
Broiled Lamb Patty, Mint Jelly — 3 oz.	Broiled Lamb Patty — 3 oz.	(LS Broiled Lamb Patty, Mint Jelly — 2 oz.)
(Diced Boiled Potato — ½ cup)		(LS Mashed Potatoes — ½ cup)
(Green Beans — ½ cup)	(Green Beans — ½ cup)	(LS Buttered Green Beans — ½ cup)
Lettuce Wedge, (Low-Calorie Dressing)	Lettuce Wedge, (Low-Calorie Dressing)	Lettuce Wedge, (Special LS Dressing)
Half Grapefruit	Half Grapefruit	Half Grapefruit
Bread — 1 slice	Bread — 1 slice	Bread — 1 slice
		(LS Butter or LS Margarine — 1 pat)
Coffee or Tea	Coffee or Tea	Coffee or Tea
(Skim Milk — 1 cup)	(Skim Milk — 1 cup)	Milk — 1 cup
Sugar — as desired		Cream — (1 tbsp. if desired)
		Sugar — as desired

DIETS MODIFIED FROM THE REGULAR MENU
(Variations from the regular menu are in parentheses)

Friday

REGULAR MENU	SOFT OR BLAND
MORNING	
Orange Juice—½ cup	Orange Juice—½ cup
OR Grapefruit Juice—½ cup	
Puffed Rice Cereal—1 cup	Puffed Rice Cereal—1 cup
OR Rolled Wheat Cereal—½ cup	
Sausage Patty—1	(Soft Cooked Egg—1)
Toast—1 slice	Toast—1 slice
Butter or Margarine—1 pat	Butter or Margarine—1 pat
Jelly—2 tsp.	Jelly—2 tsp.
Coffee or Tea	Coffee or Tea (Soft Diets)
	Decaffeinated Coffee (Bland Diets)
Milk—1 cup	Milk—1 cup
Cream and Sugar—as desired	Cream and Sugar—as desired
NOON	
Vegetable Chowder—½ cup	(Strained Vegetable Chowder—½ cup)
Crackers—2	Crackers—2
Broiled Fresh Codfish, Lemon—2 oz.	Broiled Fresh Codfish, Lemon—2 oz.
OR Smoked Thuringer, Mustard	
Hot Potato Salad—½ cup	
OR Baked Potato—1 medium	Baked Potato—1 medium
	(Parsley Buttered Carrots—½ cup)
Spring Salad, French Dressing	
OR Spiced Peach and Celery Curl Salad	(Peach Half on Lettuce, Mayonnaise)
Frosted Angel Food Cake	Frosted Angel Food Cake
OR Tangerine—1 large	
Bread—1 slice	Bread—1 slice
Butter or Margarine—2 pats	Butter or Margarine—2 pats
Coffee or Tea	Coffee or Tea (Soft Diets)
	(Milk—1 cup)
Cream and Sugar—as desired	Cream and Sugar—as desired
NIGHT	
Apricot Nectar—½ cup	Apricot Nectar—½ cup
Pot Roast of Beef—3 oz.	Pot Roast of Beef—3 oz.
OR Baked Halibut, Lemon—3 oz.	
Buttered Noodles—½ cup	Buttered Noodles—½ cup
Buttered Chopped Spinach—½ cup	Buttered Chopped Spinach—½ cup
OR Buttered Wax Beans—½ cup	
Grapefruit and Apple Salad	
OR Pickled Beet and Onion Ring Salad	
Fresh Rhubarb—½ cup	
OR Vanilla Blancmange with Chocolate Sauce	Vanilla Blancmange with Chocolate Sauce
Dinner Roll—1	Dinner Roll—1
Butter or Margarine—1 pat	Butter or Margarine—1 pat
Coffee or Tea	Coffee or Tea (Soft Diets)
Milk—1 cup	Milk—1 cup
Cream and Sugar—as desired	Cream and Sugar—as desired

DIETS MODIFIED FROM THE REGULAR MENU
(Variations from the regular menu are in parentheses)

Low Fat (35 grams fat — No fat added in cooking)	1000 Calorie (No fat or sugar added in cooking)	1000 mg. Sodium (No salt, soda, baking powder or salted fat added in cooking (including baking) or other preparation. When more than 3 slices of bread are served in a day, the extra slices must be low sodium bread. LS means low sodium. All canned vegetables should be LS.)
MORNING		
Orange Juice — ½ cup	Orange Juice — ½ cup	Orange Juice — ½ cup
Puffed Rice Cereal — 1 cup	Puffed Rice Cereal — 1 cup OR Toast — 1 slice	Puffed Rice Cereal — 1 cup
(Soft Cooked Egg — 1) Toast — 1 slice Jelly — 2 tsp.	(Soft Cooked Egg — 1)	(Soft Cooked Egg — 1) Toast — 1 slice (LS Butter or LS Margarine — 1 pat)
Coffee or Tea	Coffee or Tea	Coffee or Tea
(Skim Milk — 1 cup) Sugar — as desired	(Skim Milk — 1 cup)	Milk — 1 cup Cream — (1 tbsp. if desired) Sugar — as desired
NOON		
(Fat-Free Vegetable Chowder — ½ cup Crackers — 2 Broiled Fresh Codfish, Lemon — 2 oz. Baked Potato — 1 medium	Broiled Fresh Codfish, Lemon — 3 oz. (Parsley Carrots — ½ cup)	(LS Broiled Fresh Codfish, Lemon — 2 oz.) Baked Potato — 1 medium (LS Buttered Brussels Sprouts)
Spring Salad, (Low-Calorie Dressing) (Plain) Angel Food Cake	Spring Salad, (Low-Calorie Dressing)	Spring Salad, (Special LS Dressing)
	Tangerine — 1 large	Tangerine — 1 large Bread — 1 slice
Bread — 1 slice (Preserves — 2 tsp.) Coffee or Tea	Coffee or Tea	(LS Butter or LS Margarine — 1 pat) Coffee or Tea Cream — (1 tbsp. if desired)
Sugar — as desired		Sugar — as desired
NIGHT		
Apricot Nectar — ½ cup Pot Roast of Beef — 3 oz.	Pot Roast of Beef — 3 oz.	Apricot Nectar — ½ cup (LS Pot Roast of Beef — 2 oz.)
(Noodles — ½ cup) (Chopped Spinach — ½ cup)	(Chopped Spinach — ½ cup)	(LS Buttered Noodles — ½ cup) (LS Buttered Wax Beans — ½ cup)
Grapefruit and Apple Salad, (Low-Calorie Dressing)	(Fresh Grapefruit and Apple Salad — ½ cup, (Low-Calorie Dressing)	Grapefruit and Apple Salad, (Special LS Dressing)
Fresh Rhubarb — ½ cup	(Fresh Rhubarb, Art. Sweet. — ½ cup)	Fresh Rhubarb — ½ cup
Dinner Roll — 1 (Jelly — 2 tsp.) Coffee or Tea (Skim Milk — 1 cup) Sugar — as desired	Dinner Roll — 1 Coffee or Tea (Skim Milk — 1 cup)	Dinner Roll — 1 (LS Butter or LS Margarine — 1 pat) Coffee or Tea Milk — 1 cup Cream — (1 tbsp. if desired) Sugar — as desired

DIETS MODIFIED FROM THE REGULAR MENU
(Variations from the regular menu are in parentheses)

SATURDAY
REGULAR MENU	SOFT OR BLAND
MORNING	
Orange Quarters — 4	
OR Blended Vegetable Juice — ½ cup	Blended Vegetable Juice — ½ cup
Oatmeal — ½ cup	Oatmeal — ½ cup
OR Shredded Wheat — 1 biscuit	Crisp Bacon — 2 slices
Cinnamon Toast — 1 slice	(Toast — 1 slice)
Butter or Margarine — 1 pat	Butter or Margarine — 1 pat
Jelly — 2 tsp.	Jelly — 2 tsp.
Coffee or Tea	Coffee or Tea (Soft Diets)
	Decaffeinated Coffee (Bland Diets)
Milk — 1 cup	Milk — 1 cup
Cream and Sugar — as desired	Cream and Sugar — as desired
NOON	
Chicken Noodle Soup — ½ cup	Chicken Noodle Soup — ½ cup (Soft Diets)
Oyster Crackers	Oyster Crackers (Soft Diets)
Meatballs — 3 oz.	Meatballs — 3 oz.
OR Chicken Salad — 3 oz. (with Tomato Wedges)	
Parsley Buttered Potato — 1 medium	Parsley Buttered Potato — 1 medium
	(Buttered Green Peas — ½ cup)
Tossed Vegetable Salad, 1000 Island Dressing	
OR Lime Gelatin and Cottage Cheese Salad	Lime Gelatin and Cottage Cheese Salad
Greengage Plums in Syrup — ½ cup	
OR Rice Pudding, Raisin Sauce — ½ cup	(Rice Pudding — ½ cup)
Buttercrisp Roll — 1	Buttercrisp Roll — 1
Butter or Margarine — 1 pat	Butter or Margarine — 1 pat
Coffee or Tea	Coffee or Tea (Soft Diets)
	Milk — 1 cup (Bland Diets)
Cream and Sugar — as desired	Cream and Sugar — as desired
NIGHT	
Roast Leg of Lamb — 3 oz.	Roast Leg of Lamb — 3 oz.
OR Spanish Omelet	
Pimento Creamed Potatoes — ½ cup	(Creamed Potatoes — ½ cup)
Buttered Asparagus Spears — ½ cup	Buttered Asparagus Spears — ½ cup
OR Spiced Beets — ½ cup	
Mixed Fruit Salad	(Peach Half on Lettuce, Mayonnaise)
OR Head Lettuce, Chiffonade Dressing	
Frozen Strawberries — ½ cup	
OR Chocolate Cupcake	Chocolate Cupcake
Garlic Buttered French Bread — 1 slice	
OR Bread — 1 slice	Bread — 1 slice
Butter or Margarine — 1 pat	Butter or Margarine — 1 pat
Coffee or Tea	Coffee or Tea (Soft Diets)
Milk — 1 cup	Milk — 1 cup
Cream and Sugar — as desired	Cream and Sugar — as desired

DIETS MODIFIED FROM THE REGULAR MENU
(VARIATIONS FROM THE REGULAR MENU ARE IN PARENTHESES)

LOW FAT (35 grams fat — No fat added in cooking)	1000 CALORIE (No fat or sugar added in cooking)	1000 MG. SODIUM (No salt, soda, baking powder or salted fat added in cooking (including baking) or other preparation. When more than 3 slices of bread are served in a day, the extra slices must be low-sodium bread. LS means low sodium. All canned vegetables should be LS.)
MORNING Orange Quarters — 4	Orange Quarters — 4	Orange Quarters — 4
Oatmeal — ½ cup	Oatmeal — ½ cup OR (Toast — 1 slice)	
(Scrambled Egg — 1) (Toast — 1 slice)	Scrambled Egg — 1	Shredded Wheat — 1 biscuit (LS Scrambled Egg — 1) (Toast — 1 slice) (LS Butter or LS Margarine — 1 pat)
Jelly — 2 tsp.	Coffee or Tea	Coffee or Tea
(Skim Milk — 1 cup) Sugar — as desired	(Skim Milk — 1 cup)	Milk — 1 cup Cream — (1 tbsp. if desired) Sugar — as desired
NOON (Fat-Free Chicken Noodle Soup — ½ cup) Oyster Crackers Meatballs — (2 oz.)	(Fat-Free Chicken Broth — ½ cup) Meatballs — 3 oz.	 (LS Meatballs — 2 oz.)
(Parsley Potato — 1 medium)	(Green Peas — 1 cup)	(LS Buttered Green Peas — ½ cup) (LS Parsley Buttered Potato — 1 medium)
Tossed Vegetable Salad (Low-Calorie Dressing)	Tossed Vegetable Salad, (Low-Calorie Dressing)	Tossed Vegetable Salad, (Special LS Dressing)
Greengage Plums in Syrup — ½ cup (Bread — 1 slice) (Honey — 2 tsp.) Coffee or Tea Sugar — as desired	(Greengage Plums, Art.Sweet. — 2) Coffee or Tea	Greengage Plums in Syrup — ½ cup (Bread — 1 slice) (LS Butter or LS Margarine — 1 pat) Coffee or Tea Cream — (1 tbsp. if desired) Sugar — as desired
NIGHT Roast Leg of Lamb — 3 oz.	Roast Leg of Lamb — 3 oz.	(LS Roast Leg of Lamb — 2 oz.)
(Diced Potato — ½ cup)		(LS Pimento Creamed Potatoes — ½ cup)
(Asparagus Spears — ½ cup)	Asparagus Spears — ½ cup	(LS Buttered Asparagus Spears — ½ cup)
Mixed Fruit Salad, (Low-Calorie Dressing) Frozen Strawberries — ½ cup	Head Lettuce, (Low-Calorie Dressing) (Fresh Strawberries — 1 cup)	Mixed Fruit Salad, (Special LS Dressing) Frozen Strawberries — ½ cup
Bread — 1 slice (Jelly — 2 tsp.) Coffee or Tea Sugar — as desired	Bread — 1 slice Coffee or Tea (Skim Milk — 1 cup)	Bread — 1 slice (LS Butter or LS Margarine — 1 pat) Coffee or Tea Milk — 1 cup Cream — (1 tbsp. if desired) Sugar — as desired

DIABETIC DIETS MODIFIED FROM THE REGULAR MENU
(Variations from the regular menu are in parentheses)
NOTE VARIATION APPLICABLE TO ALL DIABETIC DIETS: SERVE NO SUGAR. ADD NO FAT OR SUGAR IN COOKING OR OTHER PREPARATION.

Sunday

Regular Menu	1200 Calorie	1500 Calorie
MORNING		
Orange Juice—½ cup	Orange Juice—½ cup	Orange Juice—½ cup
OR Grapefruit Sections—½ cup		
Corn Flakes—¾ cup		
OR Farina—½ cup		
Poached Egg—1	Poached Egg—1	Poached Egg—1
Crisp Bacon—2 slices		
Toast—1 slice	Toast—1 slice	Toast—1 slice
Butter or Margarine—1 pat	Butter or Margarine—1 pat	Butter or Margarine—1 pat
Honey—2 tsp.		
Coffee or Tea	Coffee or Tea	Coffee or Tea
Milk—1 cup	(Skim Milk—1 cup)	Milk—1 cup
Cream and Sugar—as desired	Cream—(1 oz.)	Cream—(1 oz.)
NOON		
Bouillon—1 cup	(Fat-Free Bouillon—½ cup)	Fat-Free Bouillon—½ cup)
Roast Sirloin of Beef au jus—3 oz.	Roast Sirloin of Beef—(2 oz.)	Roast Sirloin of Beef—(2 oz.)
OR Fried Chicken—4 oz.		
Mashed Potatoes	(Boiled Potato—½ cup)	(Boiled Potato—½ cup)
	(Diced Carrots—½ cup)	(Diced Carrots—½ cup)
Chef's Salad, Vinaigrette Dressing	Chef's Salad, (Low-Calorie Dressing)	Chef's Salad, (Low-Calorie Dressing)
OR Stuffed Prune Salad		
Butterscotch Sundae		
OR Canned Pineapple in Syrup— ½ cup	(Pineapple, Art. Sweet.— ½ cup)	Pineapple, Art. Sweet.— ½ cup)
Bread—1 slice		Bread—1 slice
Butter or Margarine—1 pat	Butter or Margarine—1 pat	Butter or Margarine—1 pat
Coffee or Tea	Coffee or Tea	Coffee or Tea
Cream and Sugar—as desired		
NIGHT		
Broiled Hamburger Steak, Catsup—3 oz.	Broiled Hamburger Steak— 3 oz.	Broiled Hamburger Steak— 3 oz.
OR Ham Salad, Stuffed Olives—½ cup		
Baked Potato—1 medium		Baked Potato—(1 small)
Seasoned Green Beans—½ cup	(Green Beans—½ cup)	(Green Beans—½ cup)
OR Buttered Diced Turnips—½ cup		
Coleslaw with Celery Seed Dressing	Coleslaw with Celery Seed, (Low-Calorie Dressing)	Coleslaw with Celery Seed, (Low-Calorie Dressing)
OR Pear—Mint Jelly Salad, Mayonnaise		
Canned Fruit Cup—½ cup	(Canned Fruit Cup, Art. Sweet.—½ cup)	(Canned Fruit Cup, Art. Sweet.—½ cup)
OR Banana Gelatin, Whipped Cream— ½ cup		
Bread—1 slice	Bread—1 slice	Bread—1 slice
Butter or Margarine—2 pats	Butter or Margarine—(1 pat)	Butter or Margarine—(1 pat)
Coffee or Tea	Coffee or Tea	Coffee or Tea
Milk—1 cup		
Cream and Sugar—as desired		
NIGHT NOURISHMENT		
	(Skim Milk—1 cup)	(Milk—1 cup)
	(Saltines—5)	(Saltines—5)

DIABETIC DIETS MODIFIED FROM THE REGULAR MENU
(VARIATIONS FROM THE REGULAR MENU ARE IN PARENTHESES)

NOTE VARIATION APPLICABLE TO ALL DIABETIC DIETS: SERVE NO SUGAR. ADD NO FAT OR SUGAR IN COOKING OR OTHER PREPARATION.

1800 CALORIE	2200 CALORIE	1800 CALORIE (Suitable for pregnant women and for children 9 years of age and over)
MORNING		
Orange Juice — ½ cup	Orange Juice — ½ cup	Orange Juice — ½ cup
Corn Flakes — ¾ cup	Corn Flakes — ¾ cup	
Poached Egg — 1	Poached Egg — 1	Poached Egg — 1
Toast — 1 slice	Toast — (2 slices)	Toast — 1 slice
Butter or Margarine — 1 pat	Butter or Margarine — (2 pats)	Butter or Margarine — 1 pat
Coffee or Tea	Coffee or Tea	Coffee or Tea (Adults)
Milk — 1 cup	Milk — 1 cup	Milk — 1 cup
Cream — (1 oz.)	Cream — (1 oz.)	
NOON		
(Fat-Free Bouillon — ½ cup)	(Fat-Free Bouillon — ½ cup)	(Fat-Free Bouillon — ½ cup)
Roast Sirloin of Beef — 3 oz.	Roast Sirloin of Beef — 3 oz.	Roast Sirloin of Beef — (2 oz.)
(Boiled Potato — ½ cup)	(Boiled Potato — ½ cup)	(Boiled Potato — ½ cup)
(Diced Carrots — ½ cup)	(Diced Carrots — ½ cup)	(Diced Carrots — ½ cup)
Chef's Salad, (Low-Calorie Dressing)	Chef's Salad, (Low-Calorie Dressing)	Chef's Salad, (Low-Calorie Dressing)
(Pineapple, Art. Sweet. — ½ cup)	(Pineapple, Art. Sweet. — ½ cup)	(Pineapple, Art. Sweet. — ½ cup)
Bread — 1 slice	Bread — (2 slices)	Bread — 1 slice
Butter or Margarine — 1 pat	Butter or Margarine — (2 pats)	Butter or Margarine — 1 pat
Coffee or Tea	Coffee or Tea	Coffee or Tea (Adults)
		(Milk — 1 cup)
NIGHT		
Broiled Hamburger Steak — 3 oz.	Broiled Hamburger Steak — 4 oz.	Broiled Hamburger Steak — (2 oz.)
Baked Potato — (1 small)	Baked Potato — (1 small)	Baked Potato — (1 small)
(Green Beans — ½ cup)	(Green Beans — (½ cup)	(Green Beans — ½ cup)
Coleslaw with Celery Seed, (Low-Calorie Dressing)	Coleslaw with Celery Seed, (Low-Calorie Dressing)	Coleslaw with Celery Seed, (Low-Calorie Dressing)
(Canned Fruit Cup, Art. Sweet. — ½ cup)	(Canned Fruit Cup, Art. Sweet. — ½ cup)	(Canned Fruit Cup, Art. Sweet. — ½ cup)
Bread — (2 slices)	Bread — (2 slices)	Bread — 1 slice
Butter or Margarine — 2 pats	Butter or Margarine — (3 pats)	Butter or Margarine — (1 pat)
Coffee or Tea	Coffee or Tea	Coffee or Tea (Adults)
		Milk — 1 cup
NIGHT NOURISHMENT		
(Milk — 1 cup)	(Milk — 1 cup)	(Milk — 1 cup)
(Saltines — 5)	(Saltines — 5)	(Saltines — 5)

DIABETIC DIETS MODIFIED FROM THE REGULAR MENU
(Variations from the regular menu are in parentheses)
NOTE VARIATION APPLICABLE TO ALL DIABETIC DIETS: SERVE NO SUGAR. ADD NO FAT OR SUGAR IN COOKING
OR OTHER PREPARATION.

Monday

REGULAR MENU	1200 CALORIE	1500 CALORIE
MORNING		
Orange Juice—½ cup	Orange Juice—½ cup	Orange Juice—½ cup
OR Half Grapefruit		
Farina—½ cup		
OR Dry Malt Cereal—¾ cup		
Sausage Links—2	Sausage Links—2	Sausage Links—2
Toast—1 slice	Toast—1 slice	Toast—1 slice
Butter or Margarine—1 pat		
Jelly—2 tsp.		
Coffee or Tea	Coffee or Tea	Coffee or Tea
Milk—1 cup	(Skim Milk—1 cup)	Milk—1 cup
Cream and Sugar—as desired		
NOON		
Fresh Vegetable Soup—½ cup	(Fat-Free Vegetable Soup— ½ cup)	(Fat-Free Vegetable Soup— ½ cup)
Crackers—2		
Baked Veal Steak—2 oz.	Baked Veal Steak—2 oz.	Baked Veal Steak—2 oz.
OR Broiled Canadian Bacon—2 oz.		
Parsley Buttered Potato—1 medium		(Parsley Potato—1 small)
	(Green Peas—½ cup)	(Green Peas—½ cup)
Pineapple-Marshmallow- Date Salad		
OR Celery-Cabbage Salad, French Dressing	Celery-Cabbage Salad, (Low-Calorie Dressing)	Celery-Cabbage Salad, (Low-Calorie Dressing)
Butterscotch Meringue Pudding		
OR Canned Apricot Halves in Syrup—½ cup	(Canned Apricot Halves, Art. Sweet.—4 halves)	(Canned Apricot Halves, Art. Sweet.—4 halves)
Bread—1 slice	Bread—1 slice	Bread—1 slice
Butter or Margarine—1 pat	Butter or Margarine—1 pat	Butter or Margarine—1 pat
Coffee or Tea	Coffee or Tea	Coffee or Tea
Cream and Sugar—as desired		
NIGHT		
Roast Leg of Lamb—3 oz.	Roast Leg of Lamb—3 oz.	Roast Leg of Lamb—3 oz.
OR Chicken Cutlet, Cream Sauce—4 oz.		
Whipped Potatoes—½ cup		Whipped Potatoes—½ cup
Buttered Asparagus Spears—½ cup	(Asparagus Spears—½ cup)	(Asparagus Spears—½ cup)
OR Buttered Succotash—½ cup		
Carrot and Raisin Salad	(Celery Sticks, Dill Pickle Strips—3 or 4)	(Celery Sticks, Dill Pickle Strips—3 or 4)
OR Pear-Toasted Coconut Salad, Mayonnaise		
Applesauce—½ cup	(Applesauce, Art. Sweet.—½ cup)	(Applesauce, Art. Sweet.—½ cup)
OR Blueberry Cobbler		
Parker House Roll—1	Parker House Roll—1	Parker House Roll—1
Butter or Margarine—1 pat	Butter or Margarine—1 pat	Butter or Margarine—1 pat
Coffee or Tea	Coffee or Tea	Coffee or Tea
Milk—1 cup		
Sugar and Cream—as desired		
NIGHT NOURISHMENT		
	(Skim Milk—1 cup)	(Milk—1 cup)
	(Graham Crackers—2)	(Graham Crackers—2)

DIABETIC DIETS MODIFIED FROM THE REGULAR MENU

(Variations from the regular menu are in parentheses)

NOTE VARIATION APPLICABLE TO ALL DIABETIC DIETS: SERVE NO SUGAR. ADD NO FAT OR SUGAR IN COOKING OR OTHER PREPARATION.

1800 Calorie	2200 Calorie	1800 Calorie (Suitable for pregnant women and for children 9 years of age and over)
MORNING		
Orange Juice—½ cup	Orange Juice—½ cup	Orange Juice—½ cup
Farina—½ cup	Farina—½ cup	
Sausage Links—2	Sausage Links—2	Sausage Links—2
Toast—1 slice	Toast—(2 slices)	Toast—1 slice
	Butter or Margarine—1 pat	Butter or Margarine—1 pat
Coffee or Tea	Coffee or Tea	Coffee or Tea (Adults)
Milk—1 cup	Milk—1 cup	Milk—1 cup
NOON		
(Fat-Free Vegetable Soup—½ cup)	(Fat-Free Vegetable Soup—½ cup)	(Fat-Free Vegetable Soup—½ cup)
Baked Veal Steak—(3 oz.)	Baked Veal Steak—(3 oz.)	Baked Veal Steak—2 oz.
(Parsley Potato—1 small)	(Parsley Potato—1 small)	(Parsley Potato—1 small)
(Green Peas—½ cup)	(Green Peas—½ cup)	(Green Peas—½ cup)
Celery-Cabbage Salad, (Low-Calorie Dressing)	Celery-Cabbage Salad, (Low-Calorie Dressing)	Celery-Cabbage Salad, (Low-Calorie Dressing)
(Canned Apricot Halves, Art. Sweet.—4 halves)	(Canned Apricot Halves, Art. Sweet.—4 halves)	(Canned Apricot Halves, Art. Sweet.—4 halves)
Bread—1 slice	Bread—(2 slices)	Bread—1 slice
Butter or Margarine—1 pat	Butter or Margarine—(2 pats)	Butter or Margarine—1 pat
Coffee or Tea	Coffee or Tea	Coffee or Tea (Adults)
		(Skim Milk—1 cup)
NIGHT		
Roast Leg of Lamb—3 oz.	Roast Leg of Lamb—(4 oz.)	Roast Leg of Lamb—(2 oz.)
Whipped Potatoes—½ cup	Whipped Potatoes—½ cup	Whipped Potatoes—½ cup
(Asparagus Spears—½ cup)	(Asparagus Spears—½ cup)	(Asparagus Spears—½ cup)
(Celery Sticks, Dill Pickle Strips—3 or 4)	(Celery Sticks, Dill Pickle Strips—3 or 4)	(Celery Sticks, Dill Pickle Strips—3 or 4)
(Applesauce, Art. Sweet.—½ cup)	(Applesauce, Art. Sweet.—1 cup)	(Applesauce, Art. Sweet.—½ cup)
Parker House Roll—(2)	Parker House Roll—(2)	Parker House Roll—1
Butter or Margarine—(2 pats)	Butter or Margarine—(3 pats)	Butter or Margarine—1 pat
Coffee or Tea	Coffee or Tea	Coffee or Tea (Adults)
		Milk—1 cup
NIGHT NOURISHMENT		
(Milk—1 cup)	(Milk—1 cup)	(Milk—1 cup)
(Graham Crackers—2)	(Graham Crackers—2)	(Graham Crackers—2)

DIABETIC DIETS MODIFIED FROM THE REGULAR MENU
(Variations from the regular menu are in parentheses)
NOTE VARIATION APPLICABLE TO ALL DIABETIC DIETS: SERVE NO SUGAR. ADD NO FAT OR SUGAR IN COOKING OR OTHER PREPARATION.

Tuesday REGULAR MENU	1200 Calorie	1500 Calorie
MORNING		
Half Grapefruit	Half Grapefruit	Half Grapefruit
OR Orange Juice—½ cup		
Oatmeal—½ cup		
OR Corn Flakes—¾ cup		
Soft-Cooked Egg—1	Soft Cooked Egg—1	Soft Cooked Egg—1
Crisp Bacon—2 slices	Crisp Bacon—(1 slice)	Crisp Bacon—(1 slice)
Cinnamon Roll—1	(Toast—1 slice)	(Toast—1 slice)
Butter or Margarine—1 pat	Butter or Margarine—1 pat	Butter or Margarine—1 pat
Coffee or Tea	Coffee or Tea	Coffee or Tea
Milk—1 cup	(Skim Milk—1 cup)	Milk—1 cup
Cream and Sugar—as desired		
NOON		
Beef Stew with Vegetables—5 oz.		
OR Salad Plate with Cottage Cheese, Cold Cuts and Sliced Tomato	(Salad Plate with Cottage Cheese (¼ cup), Cold Cuts (1 slice), Sliced Tomato, Low-Calorie Dressing)	(Salad Plate with Cottage Cheese (¼ cup), Cold Cuts (1 slice) Sliced Tomato, Low-Calorie Dressing)
Baked Potato—1 medium		Baked Potato—(1 small)
Peach Cup Salad, Mayonnaise	(Broccoli—½ cup)	(Broccoli—½ cup)
OR Head Lettuce Salad, French Dressing		
Pineapple Tidbits—½ cup	(Pineapple Tidbits, Art. Sweet.—½ cup)	Pineapple Tidbits, Art. Sweet.—½ cup)
OR Chocolate Brownie (no nuts)—1		
Roll—1	Roll—1	Roll—1
Butter or Margarine—2 pats	Butter or Margarine—(1 pat)	Butter or Margarine—(1 pat)
Coffee or Tea	Coffee or Tea	Coffee or Tea
Cream and Sugar—as desired		
NIGHT		
Cream of Pea Soup—½ cup		
Crackers—2		
Salisbury Steak, Catsup—3 oz.		
OR Broiled Calves' Liver, Onion Gravy—3 oz.	Broiled Calves' Liver—3 oz.	Broiled Calves' Liver—3 oz.
Buttered Rice—½ cup		(Rice—½ cup)
Buttered Sliced Beets—½ cup	(Sliced Beets—½ cup)	(Sliced Beets—½ cup)
OR Buttered Cauliflower—½ cup		
Waldorf Salad		
OR Chef's Salad, French Dressing	Chef's Salad, (Low-Calorie Dressing)	Chef's Salad, (Low-Calorie Dressing)
Cherry Shortcake, Whipped Cream		
OR Bartlett Pear Half in Syrup	(Pear Halves, Art. Sweet.—2)	(Pear Halves, Art. Sweet.—2)
Bread—1 slice	Bread—1 slice	Bread—1 slice
Butter or Margarine—1 pat	Butter or Margarine—1 pat	Butter or Margarine—1 pat
Coffee or Tea	Coffee or Tea	Coffee or Tea
Milk—1 cup		
Cream and Sugar—as desired		
NIGHT NOURISHMENT		
	(Skim Milk—1 cup)	(Milk—1 cup)
	(Graham Crackers—2)	(Graham Crackers—2)

DIABETIC DIETS MODIFIED FROM THE REGULAR MENU
(VARIATIONS FROM THE REGULAR MENU ARE IN PARENTHESES)
NOTE VARIATION APPLICABLE TO ALL DIABETIC DIETS: SERVE NO SUGAR. ADD NO FAT OR SUGAR IN COOKING OR OTHER PREPARATION.

1800 CALORIE	2200 CALORIE	1800 CALORIE (Suitable for pregnant women and for children 9 years of age and over)
MORNING		
Half Grapefruit	Half Grapefruit	Half Grapefruit
Oatmeal—½ cup	Oatmeal—½ cup	
Soft Cooked Egg—1	Soft Cooked Egg—1	Soft Cooked Egg—1
Crisp Bacon—(1 slice)	Crisp Bacon—(1 slice)	
(Toast—1 slice)	(Toast—2 slices)	(Toast—1 slice)
Butter or Margarine—1 pat	Butter or Margarine—(2 pats)	(Butter or Margarine—1 pat
Coffee or Tea	Coffee or Tea	Coffee or Tea (Adults)
Milk—1 cup	Milk—1 cup	Milk—1 cup
NOON		
(Salad Plate with Cottage Cheese (½ cup), Cold Cuts (1 slice), Sliced Tomato, Low-Calorie Dressing)	(Salad Plate with Cottage Cheese (½ cup), Cold Cuts (1 slice), Sliced Tomato, Low-Calorie Dressing)	(Salad Plate with Cottage Cheese (¼ cup), Cold Cuts (1 slice), Sliced Tomato, Low-Calorie Dressing)
Baked Potato—(1 small)	Baked Potato—(1 small)	Baked Potato—(1 small)
(Broccoli—½ cup)	(Broccoli—½ cup)	(Broccoli—½ cup)
Pineapple Tidbits, Art. Sweet.—½ cup)	Pineapple Tidbits, Art. Sweet.—½ cup)	(Pineapple Tidbits, Art. Sweet.—½ cup)
Roll—1	Rolls—(2)	Roll—1
Butter or Margarine—(1 pat)	Butter or Margarine—2 pats	Butter or Margarine—(1 pat)
Coffee or Tea	Coffee or Tea	Coffee or Tea (Adults)
		(Milk—1 cup)
NIGHT		
Broiled Calves' Liver—3 oz.	Broiled Calves' Liver—(4 oz.)	Broiled Calves' Liver—(2 oz.)
(Rice—½ cup)	(Rice—½ cup)	(Rice—½ cup)
(Sliced Beets—½ cup)	(Sliced Beets—½ cup)	(Sliced Beets—½ cup)
Chef's Salad, (Low-Calorie Dressing)	Chef's Salad, (Low-Calorie Dressing)	Chef's Salad, (Low-Calorie Dressing)
(Pear Halves, Art. Sweet.—2)	(Pear Halves, Art. Sweet.—4)	(Pear Halves, Art. Sweet.—2)
Bread—(2 slices)	Bread—(2 slices)	Bread—1 slice
Butter or Margarine—(2 pats)	Butter or Margarine—(3 pats)	Butter or Margarine—1 pat
Coffee or Tea	Coffee or Tea	Coffee or Tea (Adults)
		Milk—1 cup
NIGHT NOURISHMENT		
(Milk—1 cup)	(Milk—1 cup)	(Milk—1 cup)
(Graham Crackers—2)	(Graham Crackers—2)	(Graham Crackers—2)

DIABETIC DIETS MODIFIED FROM THE REGULAR MENU
(VARIATIONS FROM THE REGULAR MENU ARE IN PARENTHESES)
NOTE VARIATION APPLICABLE TO ALL DIABETIC DIETS: SERVE NO SUGAR. ADD NO FAT OR SUGAR IN COOKING
OR OTHER PREPARATION.

WEDNESDAY REGULAR MENU	1200 CALORIE	1500 CALORIE
MORNING		
Tomato Juice—½ cup		
OR Orange Halves—2	Orange Halves—2	Orange Halves—2
Cooked Malt Cereal—½ cup		
OR Puffed Rice—1 cup		
Grilled Ham Slice—1 oz.	Grilled Ham Slice—1 oz.	Grilled Ham Slice—1 oz.
Toast—1 slice	Toast—1 slice	Toast—1 slice
Butter or Margarine—1 pat	Butter or Margarine—1 pat	Butter or Margarine—1 pat
Coffee or Tea	Coffee or Tea	Coffee or Tea
Milk—1 cup	(Skim Milk—1 cup)	Milk—1 cup
Cream and Sugar—as desired	Cream—(1 oz.)	Cream—(1 oz.)
NOON		
Cranberry Juice Cocktail—½ cup	(Cranberry Juice Cocktail, Art. Sweet.—½ cup)	(Cranberry Juice Cocktail, Art. Sweet.—½ cup)
Broiled Perch Filet, Lemon—2 oz.	Broiled Perch Filet, Lemon—2 oz.	Broiled Perch Filet, Lemon—2 oz.
OR Roast Loin of Pork—2 oz.		
Steamed Potato in Jacket— 1 medium		Steamed Potato in Jacket— (1 small)
	(Chopped Spinach—½ cup)	(Chopped Spinach—½ cup)
Citrus Fruit Salad		
OR Assorted Relishes	Assorted Relishes	Assorted Relishes
Lime Sherbet—½ cup	(Raw Apple—1 small)	(Raw Apple—1 small)
OR Spice Cake, Maple Frosting		
Bread, Whole Wheat—1 slice	Bread, Whole Wheat—1 slice	Bread, Whole Wheat—1 slice
Butter or Margarine—2 pats	Butter or Margarine—(1 pat)	Butter or Margarine—(1 pat)
Coffee or Tea	Coffee or Tea	Coffee or Tea
Cream and Sugar—as desired		
NIGHT		
Roast Chicken—3 oz.	Roast Chicken (boned)—3 oz.	Roast Chicken (boned)—3 oz.
OR Veal Fricassee—4 oz.		
Buttered Noodles—½ cup		(Noodles—½ cup)
OR Buttered Rice—½ cup		
Scalloped Tomatoes—½ cup	(Chilled Canned Tomatoes— ½ cup)	(Chilled Canned Tomatoes— ½ cup)
OR Buttered Green Peas—½ cup	(Green Peas—½ cup)	(Green Peas—½ cup)
Melon ball Salad	(Leaf Lettuce, Low-Calorie Dressing)	(Leaf Lettuce, Low-Calorie Dressing)
OR Cottage Cheese with Chives		
Italian Prune Plums—½ cup	(Italian Prune Plums, Art. Sweet.—2)	(Italian Prune Plums, Art. Sweet.—2)
OR Floating Island		
Biscuit—1	Biscuit—1	Biscuit—1
Butter or Margarine—1 pat	Butter or Margarine—1 pat	Butter or Margarine—1 pat
Coffee or Tea	Coffee or Tea	Coffee or Tea
Milk—1 cup		
Cream and Sugar—as desired		
NIGHT NOURISHMENT		
	(Skim Milk—1 cup)	(Milk—1 cup)
	(Saltines—5)	(Saltines—5)

DIABETIC DIETS MODIFIED FROM THE REGULAR MENU
(VARIATIONS FROM THE REGULAR MENU ARE IN PARENTHESES)
NOTE VARIATION APPLICABLE TO ALL DIABETIC DIETS: SERVE NO SUGAR. ADD NO FAT OR SUGAR IN COOKING
OR OTHER PREPARATION.

1800 CALORIE	2200 CALORIE	1800 CALORIE (Suitable for pregnant women and for children 9 years of age and over)
MORNING		
Orange Halves—2	Orange Halves—2	Orange Halves—2
Cooked Malt Cereal—½ cup	Cooked Malt Cereal—½ cup	
Grilled Ham Slice—1 oz.	Grilled Ham Slice—1 oz.	Grilled Ham Slice—1 oz.
Toast—1 slice	Toast—(2 slices)	Toast—1 slice
Butter or Margarine—1 pat	Butter or Margarine—(2 pats)	Butter or Margarine—1 pat
Coffee or Tea	Coffee or Tea	Coffee or Tea (Adults)
Milk—1 cup	Milk—1 cup	Milk—1 cup
Cream—(1 oz.)	Cream—(1 oz.)	
NOON		
(Cranberry Juice Cocktail, Art. Sweet.—½ cup)	(Cranberry Juice Cocktail, Art. Sweet.—½ cup)	(Cranberry Juice Cocktail, Art. Sweet.—½ cup)
Broiled Perch Filet, Lemon—(3 oz.)	Broiled Perch Filet, Lemon—(3 oz.)	Broiled Perch Filet, Lemon—2 oz.
Steamed Potato in Jacket—(1 small)	Steamed Potato in Jacket—(1 small)	Steamed Potato in Jacket—(1 small)
(Chopped Spinach—½ cup)	(Chopped Spinach—½ cup)	(Chopped Spinach—½ cup)
Assorted Relishes	Assorted Relishes	Assorted Relishes
(Raw Apple—1 small)	(Raw Apple—1 small)	(Raw Apple—1 small)
Bread, Whole Wheat—1 slice	Bread, Whole Wheat—(2 slices)	Bread, Whole Wheat—1 slice
Butter or Margarine—(1 pat)	Butter or Margarine—2 pats	Butter or Margarine—(1 pat)
Coffee or Tea	Coffee or Tea	Coffee or Tea (Adults)
		(Milk—1 cup)
NIGHT		
Roast Chicken (boned)—3 oz.	Roast Chicken (boned)—(4 oz.)	Roast Chicken (boned)—(2 oz.)
(Noodles—½ cup)	(Noodles—½ cup)	(Noodles—½ cup)
(Chilled Canned Tomatoes—½ cup)	(Chilled Canned Tomatoes—½ cup)	(Chilled Canned Tomatoes—½ cup)
(Green Peas—½ cup)	(Green Peas—½ cup)	(Green Peas—½ cup)
(Leaf Lettuce, Low-Calorie Dressing)	(Leaf Lettuce, Low-Calorie Dressing)	(Leaf Lettuce, Low-Calorie Dressing)
(Italian Prune Plums, Art. Sweet.—2)	(Italian Prune Plums, Art. Sweet.—4)	(Italian Prune Plums, Art. Sweet.—2)
Biscuit—(2)	Biscuit—(2)	Biscuit—1
Butter or Margarine—(2 pats)	Butter or Margarine—(3 pats)	Butter or Margarine—1 pat
Coffee or Tea	Coffee or Tea	Coffee or Tea (Adults)
		Milk—1 cup
NIGHT NOURISHMENT		
(Milk—1 cup)	(Milk—1 cup)	(Milk—1 cup)
(Saltines—5)	(Saltines—5)	(Saltines—5)

DIABETIC DIETS MODIFIED FROM THE REGULAR MENU
(VARIATIONS FROM THE REGULAR MENU ARE IN PARENTHESES)
NOTE VARIATION APPLICABLE TO ALL DIABETIC DIETS: SERVE NO SUGAR. ADD NO FAT OR SUGAR IN COOKING
OR OTHER PREPARATION.

THURSDAY REGULAR MENU	1200 CALORIE	1500 CALORIE
MORNING		
Orange Juice—½ cup	Orange Juice—½ cup	Orange Juice—½ cup
OR Fresh Frozen Strawberries—½ cup		
Farina—½ cup		
OR Dry Oat Flakes—¾ cup		
Scrambled Egg—1	Scrambled Egg—1	Scrambled Egg—1
Raisin Toast—1 slice	(Toast—1 slice)	(Toast—1 slice)
Butter or Margarine—1 pat	Butter or Margarine—1 pat	Butter or Margarine—1 pat
Coffee or Tea	Coffee or Tea	Coffee or Tea
Milk—1 cup	(Skim Milk—1 cup)	Milk—1 cup
Cream and Sugar—as desired	Cream—(1 oz.)	Cream—(1 oz.)
NOON		
Baked Meat Loaf—2 oz.	Baked Meat Loaf—2 oz.	Baked Meat Loaf—2 oz.
OR Welsh Rarebit with Crisp Bacon— ½ cup on Toast Points		
Oven-Browned Potato—1 medium		Oven-Browned Potato—(1 small)
	(Mashed Baked Winter Squash— ½ cup)	(Mashed Baked Winter Squash— ½ cup)
Tomato-Cucumber Salad, Olive French Dressing	Tomato-Cucumber Salad, (Low-Calorie Dressing)	Tomato-Cucumber Salad, (Low-Calorie Dressing)
OR Fresh Fruit Salad, Mayonnaise		
Royal Anne Cherries—½ cup	(Royal Anne Cherries, Art. Sweet.—10 large)	(Royal Anne Cherries, Art. Sweet.—10 large)
Vanilla Wafers—2		
OR Peach Cobbler		
Plain Muffin—1	Plain Muffin—1	Plain Muffin—1
Butter or Margarine—1 pat	Butter or Margarine—1 pat	Butter or Margarine—1 pat
Coffee or Tea	Coffee or Tea	Coffee or Tea
Cream and Sugar—as desired		
NIGHT		
Chicken Broth with Rice—½ cup	(Fat-Free Chicken Broth— ½ cup)	(Fat-Free Chicken Broth— ½ cup)
Crackers—2		
Broiled Lamb Patty, Mint Jelly— 3 oz.	Broiled Lamb Patty—3 oz.	Broiled Lamb Patty—3 oz.
OR Ham a la King on Corn Bread—4 oz.		
Mashed Potatoes—½ cup		Mashed Potatoes—½ cup
Seasoned Green Beans—½ cup	(Green Beans—½ cup)	(Green Beans—½ cup)
OR Seasoned Shredded Cabbage— ½ cup		
Lettuce Wedge, Roquefort Dressing)	Lettuce Wedge, (Low-Calorie Dressing)	Lettuce Wedge, (Low-Calorie Dressing)
OR Molded Fruit Salad		
Half Grapefruit	Half Grapefruit	Half Grapefruit
OR Butter Pecan Ice Cream—½ cup		
Corn Bread—1 square		
OR Bread—1 slice	Bread—1 slice	Bread—1 slice
Butter or Margarine—1 pat	Butter or Margarine—1 pat	Butter or Margarine—1 pat
Coffee or Tea	Coffee or Tea	Coffee or Tea
Milk—1 cup		
Cream and Sugar—as desired		
NIGHT NOURISHMENT		
	(Skim Milk—1 cup)	(Milk—1 cup)
	(Saltines—5)	(Saltines—5)

DIABETIC DIETS MODIFIED FROM THE REGULAR MENU
(Variations from the regular menu are in parentheses)

NOTE VARIATION APPLICABLE TO ALL DIABETIC DIETS: SERVE NO SUGAR. ADD NO FAT OR SUGAR IN COOKING OR OTHER PREPARATION.

1800 Calorie	2200 Calorie	1800 Calorie (Suitable for pregnant women and for children 9 years of age and over)
MORNING		
Orange Juice—½ cup	Orange Juice—½ cup	Orange Juice—½ cup
Farina—½ cup	Farina—½ cup	
Scrambled Egg—1	Scrambled Egg—1	Scrambled Egg—1
(Toast—1 slice)	(Toast—2 slices)	(Toast—1 slice)
Butter or Margarine—1 pat	Butter or Margarine—(2 pats)	Butter or Margarine—1 pat
Coffee or Tea	Coffee or Tea	Coffee or Tea (Adults)
Milk—1 cup	Milk—1 cup	Milk—1 cup
Cream—(1 oz.)	Cream—(1 oz.)	
NOON		
Baked Meat Loaf—(3 oz.)	Baked Meat Loaf—(3 oz.)	Baked Meat Loaf—2 oz.
Oven-Browned Potato—(1 small)	Oven-Browned Potato—(1 small)	Oven-Browned Potato—(1 small)
(Mashed Baked Winter Squash—½ cup)	(Mashed Baked Winter Squash—½ cup)	(Mashed Baked Winter Squash—½ cup)
Tomato-Cucumber Salad, (Low-Calorie Dressing)	Tomato-Cucumber Salad, (Low-Calorie Dressing)	Tomato-Cucumber Salad, (Low-Calorie Dressing)
(Royal Anne Cherries, Art. Sweet.—10 large)	(Royal Anne Cherries, Art. Sweet.—10 large)	(Royal Anne Cherries, Art. Sweet.—10 large)
Plain Muffin—1	Plain Muffin—(2)	Plain Muffin—1
Butter or Margarine—1 pat	Butter or Margarine—(2 pats)	Butter or Margarine—1 pat
Coffee or Tea	Coffee or Tea	Coffee or Tea (Adults)
		(Milk—1 cup)
NIGHT		
(Fat-Free Chicken Broth—½ cup)	(Fat-Free Chicken Broth—½ cup)	(Fat-Free Chicken Broth—½ cup)
	Crackers—(3)	
Broiled Lamb Patty—3 oz.	Broiled Lamb Patty—(4 oz.)	Broiled Lamb Patty—(2 oz.)
Mashed Potatoes—½ cup	Mashed Potatoes—½ cup	Mashed Potatoes—½ cup
(Green Beans—½ cup)	(Green Beans—½ cup)	(Green Beans—½ cup)
Lettuce Wedge, (Low-Calorie Dressing)	Lettuce Wedge, (Low-Calorie Dressing)	Lettuce Wedge, (Low-Calorie Dressing)
Half Grapefruit	Half Grapefruit	Half Grapefruit
Bread—(2 slices)	Bread—(2 slices)	Bread—1 slice
Butter or Margarine—(2 pats)	Butter or Margarine—(3 pats)	Butter or Margarine—1 pat
Coffee or Tea	Coffee or Tea	Coffee or Tea (Adults)
		Milk—1 cup
NIGHT NOURISHMENT		
(Milk—1 cup)	(Milk—1 cup)	(Milk—1 cup)
(Saltines—5)	(Saltines—5)	(Saltines—5)

DIABETIC DIETS MODIFIED FROM THE REGULAR MENU
(Variations from the regular menu are in parentheses)

NOTE VARIATION APPLICABLE TO ALL DIABETIC DIETS: SERVE NO SUGAR. ADD NO FAT OR SUGAR IN COOKING
OR OTHER PREPARATION.

FRIDAY REGULAR MENU	1200 CALORIE	1500 CALORIE
MORNING		
Orange Juice—½ cup	Orange Juice—½ cup	Orange Juice—½ cup
OR Grapefruit Juice—½ cup		
Puffed Rice Cereal—1 cup		Puffed Rice Cereal—1 cup
OR Rolled Wheat Cereal—½ cup		
Sausage Patty—1	Sausage Patty—1	Sausage Patty—1
Toast—1 slice	Toast—1 slice	Toast—1 slice
Butter or Margarine—1 pat		
Jelly—2 tsp.		
Coffee or Tea	Coffee or Tea	Coffee or Tea
Milk—1 cup	(Skim Milk—1 cup)	Milk—1 cup
Cream and Sugar—as desired		
NOON		
Vegetable Chowder—½ cup		
Crackers—2		
Broiled Fresh Codfish,	Broiled Fresh Codfish,	Broiled Fresh Codfish,
. Lemon—2 oz.	Lemon—2 oz.	Lemon—2 oz.
OR Smoked Thuringer, Mustard		
Hot Potato Salad—½ cup		
OR Baked Potato—1 medium		Baked Potato—(1 small)
	(Parsley Carrots—½ cup)	(Parsley Carrots—½ cup)
Spring Salad, French Dressing	Spring Salad, (Low-Calorie Dressing)	Spring Salad, (Low-Calorie Dressing)
OR Spiced Peach and Celery Curl Salad		
Frosted Angel Food Cake		
OR Tangerine—1 large	Tangerine—1 large	Tangerine—1 large
Bread—1 slice	Bread—1 slice	Bread—1 slice
Butter or Margarine—2 parts	Butter or Margarine—(1 pat)	Butter or Margarine—(1 pat)
Coffee or Tea	Coffee or Tea	Coffee or Tea
Cream and Sugar—as desired		
NIGHT		
Apricot Nectar—½ cup		
Pot Roast of Beef—3 oz.	Pot Roast of Beef—3 oz.	Pot Roast of Beef—3 oz.
OR Baked Halibut, Lemon—3 oz.		
Buttered Noodles—½ cup		(Noodles—½ cup)
Buttered Chopped Spinach—½ cup	(Chopped Spinach—½ cup)	(Chopped Spinach—½ cup)
OR Buttered Wax Beans—½ cup		
Grapefruit and Apple Salad	(Fresh Grapefruit and Apple Salad, Low-Calorie Dressing)	(Fresh Grapefruit and Apple Salad, Low-Calorie Dressing—½ cup)
OR Pickled Beet and Onion Ring Salad		
Fresh Rhubarb—½ cup	(Rhubarb, Art. Sweet.—½ cup)	(Rhubarb, Art. Sweet.—½ cup)
OR Vanilla Blancmange with Chocolate Sauce		
Dinner Roll—1	Dinner Roll—1	Dinner Roll—1
Butter or Margarine—1 pat	Butter or Margarine—1 pat	Butter or Margarine—1 pat
Coffee or Tea	Coffee or Tea	Coffee or Tea
Milk—1 cup		
Cream and Sugar—as desired		
NIGHT NOURISHMENT		
	(Skim Milk—1 cup)	(Milk—1 cup)
	(Graham Crackers—2)	(Graham Crackers—2)

DIABETIC DIETS MODIFIED FROM THE REGULAR MENU

(VARIATIONS FROM THE REGULAR MENU ARE IN PARENTHESES)

NOTE VARIATION APPLICABLE TO ALL DIABETIC DIETS: SERVE NO SUGAR. ADD NO FAT OR SUGAR IN COOKING OR OTHER PREPARATION.

1800 CALORIE	2200 CALORIE	1800 CALORIE (Suitable for pregnant women and for children 9 years of age and over)
MORNING		
Orange Juice — ½ cup	Orange Juice — ½ cup	Orange Juice — ½ cup
	Puffed Rice Cereal — 1 cup	
Sausage Patty — 1	Sausage Patty — 1	Sausage Patty — 1
Toast — 1 slice	Toast — (2 slices)	Toast — 1 slice
	Butter or Margarine — 1 pat	Butter or Margarine — 1 pat
Coffee or Tea	Coffee or Tea	Coffee or Tea (Adults)
Milk — 1 cup	Milk — 1 cup	(Skim Milk — 1 cup)
NOON		
Broiled Fresh Codfish, Lemon — (3 oz.)	Broiled Fresh Codfish, Lemon — (3 oz.)	Broiled Fresh Codfish, Lemon — 2 oz.
Baked Potato — (1 small)	Baked Potato — (1 small)	Baked Potato — (1 small)
(Parsley Carrots — ½ cup)	(Parsley Carrots — ½ cup)	(Parsley Carrots — ½ cup)
Spring Salad, (Low-Calorie Dressing)	Spring Salad, (Low-Calorie Dressing)	Spring Salad, (Low-Calorie Dressing)
Tangerine — 1 large	Tangerine — 1 large	Tangerine — 1 large
Bread — 1 slice	Bread — (2 slices)	Bread — 1 slice
Butter or Margarine — (1 pat)	Butter or Margarine — 2 pats	Butter or Margarine — (1 pat)
Coffee or Tea	Coffee or Tea	Coffee or Tea (Adults)
		(Milk — 1 cup)
NIGHT		
Pot Roast of Beef — 3 oz.	Pot Roast of Beef — (4 oz.)	Pot Roast of Beef — (2 oz.)
(Noodles — ½ cup)	(Noodles — ½ cup)	(Noodles — ½ cup)
(Chopped Spinach — ½ cup)	(Chopped Spinach — ½ cup)	(Chopped Spinach — ½ cup)
(Fresh Grapefruit and Apple Salad, (Low-Calorie Dressing — ½ cup)	(Fresh Grapefruit and Apple Salad, Low-Calorie Dressing — ½ cup)	(Fresh Grapefruit and Apple Salad, Low-Calorie Dressing — ½ cup)
(Rhubarb, Art. Sweet. — ½ cup)	(Rhubarb, Art. Sweet. — ½ cup)	(Rhubarb, Art. Sweet. — ½ cup)
Dinner Rolls — (2)	Dinner Rolls — (2)	Dinner Roll — 1
Butter or Margarine — (2 pats)	Butter or Margarine — (3 pats)	Butter or Margarine — 1 pat
Coffee or Tea	Coffee or Tea	Coffee of Tea (Adults)
		Milk — 1 cup
NIGHT NOURISHMENT		
(Milk — 1 cup)	(Milk — 1 cup)	(Milk — 1 cup)
(Graham Crackers — 2)	(Graham Crackers — 2)	(Graham Crackers — 2)

DIABETIC DIETS MODIFIED FROM THE REGULAR MENU
(VARIATIONS FROM THE REGULAR MENU ARE IN PARENTHESES)
NOTE VARIATION APPLICABLE TO ALL DIABETIC DIETS: SERVE NO SUGAR. ADD NO FAT OR SUGAR IN COOKING
OR OTHER PREPARATION.

SATURDAY REGULAR MENU	1200 CALORIE	1500 CALORIE
MORNING		
Orange Quarters—4	Orange Quarters—4	Orange Quarters—4
OR Blended Vegetable Juice—½ cup		
Oatmeal—½ cup		
OR Shredded Wheat—1 biscuit	(Scrambled Egg—1)	(Scrambled Egg—1)
Crisp Bacon—2 slices	Crisp Bacon—(1 slice)	Crisp Bacon—(1 slice)
Cinnamon Toast—1 slice	(Toast—1 slice)	(Toast—1 slice)
Butter or Margarine—1 pat	Butter or Margarine—1 pat	Butter or Margarine—1 pat
Jelly—2 tsp.		
Coffee or Tea	Coffee or Tea	Coffee or Tea
Milk—1 cup	(Skim Milk—1 cup)	Milk—1 cup
Cream and Sugar—as desired		
NOON		
Chicken Noodle Soup—½ cup	(Fat-Free Chicken Broth— ½ cup)	(Fat-Free Chicken Broth— ½ cup)
Oyster Crackers		
Meatballs—3 oz.	Meatballs—(2 oz.)	Meatballs—(2 oz.)
OR Chicken Salad, Tomato Wedges— 3 oz.		
Parsley Buttered Potato—1 medium		(Parsley Potato—1 small)
	(Green Peas—½ cup)	(Green Peas—½ cup)
Tossed Vegetable Salad, 1000 Island Dressing	Tossed Vegetable Salad, (Low-Calorie Dressing)	Tossed Vegetable Salad, (Low-Calorie Dressing)
OR Lime Gelatin and Cottage Cheese Salad		
Greengage Plums in Syrup— ½ cup	(Greengage Plums, Art. Sweet.—2)	(Greengage Plums, Art. Sweet.—2)
OR Rice Pudding, Raisin Sauce—½ cup		
Buttercrisp Roll—1	(Bread—1 slice)	(Bread—1 slice)
Butter or Margarine—1 pat	Butter or Margarine—1 pat	Butter or Margarine—1 pat
Coffee or Tea	Coffee or Tea	Coffee or Tea
Cream and Sugar—as desired		
NIGHT		
Roast Leg of Lamb—3 oz.	Roast Leg of Lamb—3 oz.	Roast Leg of Lamb—3 oz.
OR Spanish Omelette		
Pimento Creamed Potatoes—½ cup		(Diced Potato—½ cup)
Buttered Asparagus Spears—½ cup	(Asparagus Spears—½ cup)	(Asparagus Spears—½ cup)
OR Spiced Beets—½ cup		
Mixed Fruit Salad		
OR Head Lettuce, Chiffonade Dressing	Head Lettuce, (Low-Calorie Dressing)	Head Lettuce, (Low-Calorie Dressing)
Frozen Strawberries—½ cup	(Fresh Strawberries—1 cup)	(Fresh Strawberries—1 cup)
OR Chocolate Cupcake		
Garlic-Buttered French Bread— 1 slice		
OR Bread—1 slice	Bread—1 slice	Bread—1 slice
Butter or Margarine—1 pat	Butter or Margarine—1 pat	Butter or Margarine—1 pat
Coffee or Tea	Coffee or Tea	Coffee or Tea
Milk—1 cup		
Cream and Sugar—as desired		
NIGHT NOURISHMENT		
	(Skim Milk—1 cup)	(Milk—1 cup)
	(Graham Crackers—2)	(Graham Crackers—2)

DIABETIC DIETS MODIFIED FROM THE REGULAR MENU
(VARIATIONS FROM THE REGULAR MENU ARE IN PARENTHESES)
NOTE VARIATION APPLICABLE TO ALL DIABETIC DIETS: SERVE NO SUGAR. ADD NO FAT OR SUGAR IN COOKING OR OTHER PREPARATION.

1800 CALORIE	2200 CALORIE	1800 CALORIE (Suitable for pregnant women and for children 9 years of age and over)
Orange Quarters — 4	Orange Quarters — 4	Orange Quarters — 4
Oatmeal — ½ cup	Oatmeal — ½ cup	
	(Scrambled Egg — 1)	(Scrambled Egg — 1)
Crisp Bacon — (1 slice)	Crisp Bacon — (1 slice)	
(Toast — 1 slice)	(Toast — 2 slices)	(Toast — 1 slice)
Butter or Margarine — 1 pat	Butter or Margarine — (2 pats)	Butter or Margarine — 1 pat
Coffee or Tea	Coffee or Tea	Coffee or Tea (Adults)
Milk — 1 cup	Milk — 1 cup	Milk — 1 cup
NOON		
(Fat-Free Chicken Broth — ½ cup)	(Fat-Free Chicken Broth — ½ cup)	(Fat-Free Chicken Broth — ½ cup)
Meatballs — 3 oz.	Meatballs — 3 oz.	Meatballs — (2 oz.)
(Parsley Potato — 1 small)	(Parsley Potato — 1 small)	(Parsley Potato — 1 small)
(Green Peas — ½ cup)	(Green Peas — ½ cup)	(Green Peas — ½ cup)
Tossed Vegetable Salad, (Low-Calorie Dressing)	Tossed Vegetable Salad, (Low-Calorie Dressing)	Tossed Vegetable Salad, (Low-Calorie Dressing)
(Greengage Plums, Art. Sweet. — 2)	(Greengage Plums, Art. Sweet. — 2)	(Greengage Plums, Art. Sweet. — 2)
(Bread — 1 slice)	(Bread — 2 slices)	(Bread — 1 slice)
Butter or Margarine — 1 pat	Butter or Margarine — (2 pats)	Butter or Margarine — 1 pat
Coffee or Tea	Coffee or Tea	Coffee or Tea (Adults)
		(Milk — 1 cup)
NIGHT		
	(Grapefruit Juice — ½ cup)	
Roast Leg of Lamb — 3 oz.	Roast Leg of Lamb — (4 oz.)	Roast Leg of Lamb — (2 oz.)
(Diced Potato — ½ cup)	(Diced Potato — ½ cup)	(Diced Potato — ½ cup)
(Asparagus Spears — ½ cup)	(Asparagus Spears — ½ cup)	(Asparagus Spears — ½ cup)
Head Lettuce, (Low-Calorie Dressing)	Head Lettuce, (Low-Calorie Dressing)	Head Lettuce, (Low-Calorie Dressing)
(Fresh Strawberries — 1 cup)	(Fresh Strawberries — 1 cup)	(Fresh Strawberries — 1 cup)
Bread — (2 slices)	Bread — (2 slices)	Bread — 1 slice
Butter or Margarine — (2 pats)	Butter or Margarine — (3 pats)	Butter or Margarine — 1 pat
Coffee or Tea	Coffee or Tea	Coffee or Tea (Adults)
		Milk — 1 cup
NIGHT NOURISHMENT		
(Milk — 1 cup)	(Milk — 1 cup)	(Milk — 1 cup)
(Graham Crackers — 2)	(Graham Crackers — 2)	(Graham Crackers — 2)

CHAPTER SEVEN

RESTORATIVE SERVICES

Restorative (rehabilitative) services must be provided upon written order of the physician. The physician must indicate anticipated goals and is responsible for the general medical direction of such services as part of the total care of the patient. The physician must prescribe the modalities to be used and must specify the frequency of physical and occupational therapy. In addition, restorative nursing care designed to maintain function or improve the patient's ability to carry out the activities of daily living must be provided by the extended care facility.

PHYSICAL THERAPY

Patients with many kinds of diseases and conditions benefit from physical therapy. Patients with cerebral vascular accidents, cardiac problems, diabetic amputations, arthritis, low back disorders, neurological diseases, congenital anomalies and accidents of all types, including severe burns, have the greatest physical therapy needs.

The objectives of physical therapy are as follows:

To obtain certain kinds of information needed for diagnosis, therapy or evaluation of patients with certain types of illnesses and disabilities.

To prevent or minimize residual physical disabilities.

To return individuals to optimum conditions of living within their capabilities.

To accelerate convalescence and reduce the length of stay in the extended care facility.

The techniques of physical therapy include manual and electrical muscle examination, sensory and circulatory tests and measurements of range of motion. Carefully developed therapeutic exercise programs, "muscle education" and re-education in gait and functional training are used to guide patients in a program to prevent disability and to encourage progress toward a greater degree of functional independence.

The physical therapy service requires medical direction. A physician, preferably one knowledgeable or trained in the field of physiatry should be appointed to give medical guidance to the physical therapy service, to determine and interpret medical policies, to review equipment needs and to interpret and relate the physical therapy service to other medical services.

PHYSICAL THERAPIST

A qualified physical therapist is a person who graduated (after 1936) from a school or course approved by the Council on Medical Education of the American Medical Association, who graduated (prior to 1936) from a school or course approved by American Physical Therapy Association; or who is a member of the American Physical Therapy Association or registrant of the American Registry of Physical Therapists.

The physical therapist is concerned with the disabled and potentially handicapped patient. His main activities are directed toward relieving pain, preventing disability, developing or improving skills, restoring function and maintaining maximum performance within the patient s capabilities.

Non-Professional Assistant

A non-professional assistant working under the direction of the physical therapist can serve the following duties:

Act as receptionist, record patient appointments and attendance, transcribe dictated notes of the physician or physical therapist, maintain files, type reports and correspondence, requisition supplies and perform other clerical duties.

Assemble equipment and supplies needed for treatments. Keep equipment clean, properly stored, ready for use; set up apparatus and equipment such as whirlpool therapy, paraffin bath, hot packs; maintain linen supply.

Prepare patients for treatment. Assist in dressing and moving about, handle the timing of treatments, perform simple routines applying to the particular needs of the individual, transport patients to and from the treatment area.

Administration

Patients are accepted only on referral from physicians and the treatments are prescribed only by physicians.

REPORTS AND RECORDS

Narrative reports should cover such items as coordination of physical therapy with other services, additions to or reduction in staff, new equipment and goals for future development. Statistical reports should be prepared regularly.

Physical therapy record form should be consistent with the form of other medical records of the facility. Treatment records include the physician's signed prescription, progress notes, results of special tests and measurements and the patient's attendance record.

Physician's Prescription

It is imperative that the prescription be signed by the referring physician and that it include the following data: date, medical record number, patient's name, address, bed location, age, diagnosis and treatment desired. Results to be accomplished, number and frequency of treatments desired, precautions or special instructions and date of return examination or re-evaluation for changes in prescription must also be included.

Progress Notes by the Physical Therapist

Progress notes must be written at stated intervals, dated and signed by the physical therapist, kept current and made available to the referring physician. The initial note should include the patient's identifying information, initial physical therapy evaluation and treatment plan and objectives. Subsequent notes should include the patient's progress or lack thereof, symptoms noted, prescribed changes in treatment plans and devices, adaptive equipment or appliances used and the patient's proficiency in using them. Results of tests and measurements must also be included. At the time of discharge there should be a final re-evaluation related to the initial one and a summary of the course of treatment, including the reason for its termination.

Special Tests and Measurements

Results of special tests and measurements should be kept on separate, specifically designed forms to facilitate interpretation of the tests. Records of muscle tests, range of joint motion, functional activities progress and the like should be included.

Attendance Records

Each visit of the patient should be recorded and the total number of visits included in his treatment record.

Bedside Card

A record of physical therapy status is useful at the bedside for the attending physician, nurses, and others responsible for bedside care. The card should show what equipment the patient uses — wheelchair, crutches, braces — and the amount and type of assistance he needs to perform activities of daily living.

Abbreviations or symbols are to be discouraged in recording information.

PHYSICAL THERAPY UNIT

The essential components of a satisfactory physical therapy unit are as follows:

Reception area. Safe, comfortable waiting space for patients, including those in wheelchairs and on stretchers, must be provided.

Examination area. Floor-to-ceiling partitions must be installed for privacy. Examination equipment should remain in the examination room permanently. This space may also be used for giving special tests or taking measurements or for treatments.

Treatment areas. Three types of treatment areas should be designed to meet the requirements for giving various types of treatments: cubicles, hydrotherapy area and open exercise area. Each cubicle must be large enough to permit the physical therapist to work on either side of the table.

In addition, suitable office space for confidential interviewing and administrative and clerical duties is necessary. Separate toilet facilities must be available for patients and staff; and accessible, adequate, well-lighted storage space is essential. Wheelchairs, stretchers and other large, movable equipment should be stored in special areas rather than in closets.

PLANS FOR PHYSICAL THERAPY

The facility should set aside appropriate space to be used for physical therapy–related activities. The room should be esthetically pleasant and possibly have an FM radio available for background music. (Refer to Table 7–1 for basic equipment suggestions.)

The consulting physical therapist may be paid a flat contracted sum, by the hour or per patient treatment. Payment by the hour (or part-time salary) makes possible generalized consultation services which would have a beneficial effect on all residents of the facility, not only on those receiving direct treatment. Also, this method of payment is more conducive to the teaching of simple but effective rehabilitation techniques which could be regularly carried out by staff other than the physical therapist, thus enhancing the beneficial effects of the physical therapist's services.

PHYSICAL THERAPIST—POSITION SUMMARY

A registered physical therapist should be in charge of the physical therapy department. It is the responsibility of the physical therapist to interpret and implement physicians' orders regarding therapy to patients and to ensure that these orders are carried out in a professional manner. An evaluation of the rehabilitation potential of the patient should be provided by the therapist, and the goals of rehabilitation for the patient should be noted. The therapist should conduct an in-service training program for nursing personnel in order that they become aware of physical therapy and restorative services and able to participate in aiding the physical therapist in exercising patients and other forms of therapy which have been ordered. The physical therapist should participate in staff meetings and take part in the planning and budgeting for equipment, materials and supplies for the department.

QUALIFICATIONS

Graduate of a program of physical therapy approved by the Council on Medical Education of the American Medical Association in collaboration with the American Physical Therapy Association.

TABLE 7–1. PHYSICAL THERAPY

Area or Type of Equipment	PATIENT LOAD PER DAY	
	10–20	20–30
Cubicle—treatment table, footstool, chair	3	5
Examining Room—includes equipment for tests, measurements	1	1
Electrotherapy Equipment		
Infrared	1	1
Ultra Violet—general and spot	1	1
High Frequency—diathermy or microwave	1	1
Low Voltage—therapeutic and/or diagnostic	1	1
Hydrotherapy Equipment		
Hot-pack unit	1	2
Cold-pack unit	1	1
Paraffin-bath unit	1	1
Whirlpool with chair—hip, leg, arm	1	1
Therapist's stool with casters	1	1
Hand table, chair	1	1
Equipment for Other Modalities		
Tilt table	1	1
Traction	1	1
Ultrasonic	1	1
Exercise Equipment		
Mats—on floor and on platform	1	1
Parallel bars, adjustable height and width	1	2
Posture mirrors	2	2
Canes—adjustable, quadruped	1	1
Crutches, adjustable—small, medium, large	1 ea.	1 ea.
Walker	1	2
Finger ladder	1	1
Therapist's stool	1	1
Hand table and chair	1	1
Steps	1	1
Ramp, curb, stall bars	optional	
Pulleys—with weights and without weights	1 ea.	1 ea.
Shoulder wheel	1	1
General Equipment		
Interval timer	4	6
Stopwatch	1	1
Stethoscope	1	1
Sphygmomanometer	1	1
Reflex hammer	1	1
Spirometer	1	1
Endotracheal tube	1	1
First aid kit	1	1
Portable patient lift	1	1
Wheelchairs	1	2
Stretcher	1	1
Pillows, soiled linen container, waste baskets, urinals, bedpans, emesis basin, container for lubricating alcohol	as needed	
Optional Equipment		
Exercise pool		
Hair dryer		
High voltage stimulator		
Moist air unit		

PRESCRIPTION FORM — PHYSICAL THERAPY

```
NAME OF FACILITY                          PATIENT INFORMATION
ADDRESS                                   (include name, address, sex,
TELEPHONE NUMBER                          record number, room number)
PRESCRIPTION FOR PHYSICAL THERAPY
  Diagnosis,Precautions,Special Instructions.
PART(s) TO BE TREATED:_____     __Check if patient to be treated at bedside.
```

FREQUENCY OF TREATMENT
__Daily for _____ days.   __Twice weekly for _____ weeks
__Twice daily for __ days.   __Once weekly for _____ weeks
__Three times week for ___ weeks.   __Other (specify)_____

DATE OF REEXAMINATION:
TREATMENT TO BE GIVEN (list below may be checked off if such procedure has been established.
DATE_____ PHYSICIAN'S SIGNATURE _____

PHYSICAL THERAPY SERVICES

__THERAPEUTIC EXERCISE-General   __HEAT
__Passive   __Short-wave diathermy or microwave (deep,
__Active   high frequency)
__Resistive   __Infrared(radiant lamp,superficial dry)
__Progressive resistive   __Paraffin(oily,low heat conduction)
__Postural   __Baker(luminous,incandescent,superficial)
__Underwater   __Hydrocollator(pack type,moist,superficial)

__THERAPEUTIC EXERCISE-Specific   __COLD
__Codman   __Pack type,moist, short application
__Buerger   __Other (specify)_____
__Williams
__Respiratory   __HYDROTHERAPY
__Cardiac   __Hubbard tub(with or without exercise,full
__Ambulation   body immersion)
  __Prosthetic training   __Whirlpool (arm,leg,full body if sitting)
  __Gait training-with ambulatory   __Contrast bath(times,alternating hot and cold)
      aids-without aids
__Other (specify)_____   __TRACTION
                                            __Intermittent cervical,sitting or supine
__TESTS AND MEASUREMENTS   __Intermittent pelvic,supine,counter-trunk
__Manual muscle test   traction
__Electrodiagnostic(List those avail-
    able,i.e.,chronaxie,strength dura-   __ELECTROTHERAPY
    tion curves)   __Electrical stimulation(galvanic,faradic)
__Electromyograph
__Nerve conduction time study   __ULTRASOUND
__Goniometric range of motion
    measurement   __ULTRAVIOLET
__Postural analysis
__Functional activity   __MASSAGE
__Crutch measurement   __HOME INSTRUCTION
                                          __HOME VISIT(for evaluation,treatment or
                                              instruction)

                        ATTENDANCE RECORD
```

| MONTH | 1 | 2 | 3 | 4 | 5 | 6 | 7 | 8 | 9 | 10 | 11 | 12 | 13 | 14 | 15 | 16 | 17 | 18 | 19 | 20 | 21 | 22 | 23 | 24 | 25 | 26 | 27 | 28 | 29 | 30 | 31 | |
|---|---|---|---|---|---|---|---|---|---|---|---|---|---|---|---|---|---|---|---|---|---|---|---|---|---|---|---|---|---|---|---|---|
| | | | | | | | | | | | | | | | | | | | | | | | | | | | | | | | | | |
| | | | | | | | | | | | | | | | | | | | | | | | | | | | | | | | | | |
| | | | | | | | | | | | | | | | | | | | | | | | | | | | | | | | | | |

(Reverse side or separate sheet may be used for progress notes)

Be licensed as a Registered Physical Therapist in the state.

Have had one or more years of experience in a medical institution.

Be knowledgeable of standards and procedures.

Possess leadership ability to direct ancillary personnel in aiding and assisting patients in physical therapy.
```

DUTIES

Perform a physical status evaluation on all patients under the orders of the attending physician.

In cooperation with the attending physician, plan and implement a program of physical therapy for all patients.

Supervise the scheduling and execution of treatments.

Provide for evaluation of patient's status and progress.

Maintain physical therapy section of the medical record in regard to the program of therapy ordered by the attending physician.

Complete the progress forms.

Respect the confidentiality of information regarding patients.

Integrate the activities of the physical therapy department with those of other departments of the hospital.

Plan and provide for the use of equipment and materials within the space allocated.

Be responsible for recommendations for purchase and care of equipment, materials and supplies required for the operation of the department.

Cooperate with the administration in the procurement of satisfactory equipment.

Establish a program of safety in the care and treatment of patients in relation to use of equipment.

Provide for evaluation of the activities of daily living of all patients, under the direction of the attending physician.

Instruct patients and nursing personnel in self-help in the use of prosthetic devices.

Record physical therapy consultation notes in the medical records of indicated patients.

Participate in in-service training programs, both within the physical therapy department and in cooperation with other departments in the organization.

Be familiar with advances in physical therapy through literature and attendance at meetings, seminars and workshops.

OCCUPATIONAL THERAPY

Occupational therapy is given or supervised by a therapist who is registered by American Occupational Therapy Association or is a graduate of a program approved by the Council on Medical Education of the American Medical Association in collaboration with the American Occupational Therapy Association or by a therapist who is in the process of accumulating supervised clinical experience required for registration.

Occupational therapy includes duties such as assisting the physician in his evaluation of the patient's level of function by applying diagnostic and prognostic tests and guiding the patient in his use of therapeutic creative and self-care activities. All therapists must collaborate with the facility's medical and nursing staff in developing the patient's total plan of care, and all must participate in the facility's in-service education program.

AMBULATION AND THERAPEUTIC EQUIPMENT

Recommended ambulation equipment includes such items as parallel bars, hand rails, wheelchairs, walkers, walkerettes, crutches and canes. The therapist must advise the administrator concerning the purchase, rental, storage and maintenance of equipment and supplies.

OCCUPATIONAL THERAPY INITIAL EVALUATION

Patient's Name_____ Eval. Date_____ Request Date_____

Room:_____ Age:_____ Sex:_____ Referring Physician_____

Diagnosis:_____

Special Problems:_____

I. TESTS ADMINISTERED   RESULTS

_____

_____

_____

_____

II. GENERAL ABILITIES EVALUATION:
   A. Following instructions (oral, written):
   B. Learning Speed:
   C. Attention Span:
   D. Interest Level:

III. PHYSICAL EVALUATION:
   A. Range of Motion:
   B. Muscle Strength:
   C. Hand Function:
   D. Perception:
      1. Position Sense:
      2. Sensation:
      3. Stereognosis:
      4. Body Orientation:
      5. Vision:
      6. Hearing:
   E. Functional Status:

IV. SOCIAL CONSCIOUSNESS:
   A. Grooming:
   B. Self-confidence:
   C. Cooperativeness:
   D. Interaction with other patients:

V. RECOMMENDATIONS:
   A. Physical:
   B. Self-Care:
   C. Coordination training:
   D. Development of work tolerance:
   E. Interest Exploration:
   F. Supportive programming:
   G. Adapted equipment necessary

VI. OTHER COMMENTS:

_____

Evaluating Therapist

FUNCTIONAL STATUS CHART

Patient's Name _____   Address _____

FUNCTIONAL STATUS PROFILE

Mobility						
Dressing						
Eating						
Hygiene						
Toileting						
Elimination						

Instructions

The patient's present functional status should be scored (prior to evaluation or re-evaluation), not his ability or potential. If the patient seems to fall between two levels, score him at the lower level.

After determining the functional level which best describes the patient in each of the six areas, record the corresponding numbers in the appropriate places on the Function Status Profile.

MOBILITY
1. Does not move self in bed. May roll partially to one side or the other, may maintain side-lying position if so placed, or may sit in arm chair when placed there.

2. Shifts in bed from side to side and/or head to foot, and rolls from side to side. May turn over or attain partial sitting position, or may sit and balance briefly when placed in sitting position.

3. Rises to sitting position on side of bed and maintains balance well. May transfer, roll wheel chair or walk short distances with assistance.

4. Transfers with or without supervision but without assistance and rolls wheel chair. May walk with assistance and/or close supervision.

5. Transfers into and propels wheel chair without assistance or supervision; manages brakes, footrests and other attachments. May walk without assistance but with some supervision.

6. Walks independently without supervision or assistance. May or may not use apparatus (braces, crutches, canes, walker).

DRESSING
1. Dependent in all dressing activities.   )   Underline independent activities

2. Performs independently one or two of the)   a. shoes
   dressing activities.   )   b. socks
                                                        c. shirt, blouse or pajama top
3. Performs independently three or four of)____)d. trousers, skirt or pajama bottom
   the dressing activities.   )   e. slip-over garment (sweater, dress
                                                            or gown)
4. Performs independently five or six of the)   f. fastenings
   dressing activities.   )   g. undergarments

5. Performs independently all dressing activities (day and night clothing) but requires clothing to be brought to him and/or replaced.

6. Assembles and replaces all clothing (from drawers, closets, et cetera), and puts on and removes all clothing. May or may not include outer clothing (overcoat, hat, gloves).

FUNCTIONAL STATUS CHART — Continued

EATING

1. Dependent in all eating activities.

2. Finger feeds (bread, cookies, etc.). May assist minimally in eating and/or drinking.

3. Eats and drinks using utensils with some assistance.

4. Performs eating activities independently when food is prepared on plate.

5. Performs eating activities independently; takes food from table to mouth with utensil, cuts meat, butters bread, drinks liquids, reaches and uses salt shaker.

HYGIENE

1. Dependent in all hygiene activities.   )   Underline independent activities

2. Performs independently <u>one or two of</u>   )   a. washes face and hands
    the hygiene activities.   )_____)b. brushes teeth and/or dentures
                                                            c. combs or brushes hair
3. Performs independently three or four   )   d. shaves or applies make-up
    of the hygiene activities, but requires)   (if applicable)
    assistance with a complete bath.

4. Performs independently all applicable hygiene activities including complete bath but requires assistance in getting and/or putting away equipment.

5. Performs independently in all applicable activities.

TOILETING

1. Dependent in all toileting activities.   )   Underline independent activities

2. Performs independently one of the   )   a. mobility (getting to or onto bed
    toileting activities.   )_____)   pan, commode or toilet)

3. Performs independently <u>two</u> of the   )   b. clothing adjustment
    toileting activities.   )   c. cleaning self

4. Performs independently (without assistance or supervision) all toileting activities.

NOTE: The "toileting" score indicates a level of motor function.
       The "elimination" score indicates a level of physiological function.

ELIMINATION

1. <u>Incontinent of bowel and bladder</u>. Lacks control of elimination. Use of a catheter is considered incontinence.

2. <u>Incontinent of)   )</u> bowel   Underline the term that is appropriate.
                                bladder

3. <u>Incontinent of bowel and/or bladder at night</u> or has occasional accidents during the day.

4. <u>Continent</u>. Has control of elimination at all times. If patient can control his bowel or bladder function by mechanical means he should be rated as continent of that function.

OCCUPATIONAL THERAPIST—POSITION SUMMARY

QUALIFICATIONS

Education. A qualified occupational therapist is a graduate of an occupational therapy program approved by the council on medical education of the American Medical Association, in collaboration with the American Occupational Therapy Association.

Registration. The qualified occupational therapist has successfully written the registration examination given by the American Occupational Therapy Association and is currently registered by that association. In addition, it is desirable that he be a member of state and local associations.

Experience. It is preferred that the occupational therapist have had one or two years' work experience under the supervision of an experienced, qualified occupational therapist in a hospital, rehabilitation center or community agency.

Essential requirements:

A thorough knowledge of the principles and practices of occupational therapy as well as new developments in the field, plus the ability to apply them in developing a program in an extended care facility or community agency.

A thorough knowledge of state and federal standards and regulations as they apply to a particular facility or agency.

A knowledge of occupational therapy equipment and materials and their sources of supply.

A knowledge of teaching methods and the ability to demonstrate occupational therapy techniques to assistants, nurses, nurses' aides and home health aides.

The ability to establish and maintain effective working relationships with physicians, administrators, other therapists, nurses, activity supervisors and other personnel in the facility or agency.

The ability to speak effectively before groups.

A knowledge of the community and its resources.

The registered occupational therapist is administratively supervised from within the facility or agency. He receives clinical supervision from the referring physician and/or supervising occupational therapist; all matters pertaining to the occupational therapy treatment of a patient are referred to this physician and/or supervising occupational therapist.

DUTIES

Direct service is performed only on referral by a physician and continued only with medical supervision. The registered occupational therapist performs the following functions:

Assists the physician in evaluating the patient's level of function and in determining his abilities and inabilities by appropriate tests and procedures.

Assists and supports the nursing staff in carrying out the treatment plan.

Guides the patient in his use of therapeutic, creative and self-care activities to develop, restore and maintain the highest level of function.

Teaches and supervises selected occupational therapy techniques and maintenance activities to patients, family members, homemaker-home health aides, nurses' aides or other personnel to be carried on between treatments.

Plans and suggests adapted equipment and adaptations to the home environment to assist the patient to function at his highest level.

Observes (and records in the current patient record) the patient's reaction to treatment and any changes in the patient's condition. This information is also discussed with the supervising nurse and is reported to the physician where applicable.

Consultation and teaching

Assists the staff of the facility to develop their philosophy of rehabilitation and encourages its implementation.

Interprets the role of occupational therapy, general rehabilitation procedures and activity programing to physicians, administrators, nursing personnel, volunteers, etc.

Participates in staff meetings regarding patient status, patient motivation and interdepartmental communications.

Advises the home or agency regarding purchase or acquisition of equipment and supplies. The occupational therapist also advises about specific location of activities and the remodeling of areas for activities.

Provides in-service education regarding activities of daily living, general rehabilitation techniques, etc., and assists in the development of educational materials.

Strengthens the community of patient care between hospitals and related facilities and agencies through communication and planning between therapists and other personnel.

Assists the facility in developing job descriptions, procedures and rules for the occupational therapist, activity supervisor and volunteers.

Maintains a liaison with the state department of public health, occupational therapy organizations and allied professional groups.

Writes a report of consultation visits, including persons seen, subjects discussed, recommendations and subjects for future sessions. (This is a confidential report and is used only at the discretion of the occupational therapy consultant and the administrator.)

Meets regularly with the activity supervisor to plan and review the activity program and patient participation record. The purpose is to determine the effectiveness of the programing for the total patient census and to assure that individual patient needs are being met.

Evaluates patients and makes recommendations regarding general rehabilitation techniques, motivation and participation in the activity program regarding these patients.

Counsels the activity supervisor regarding the use of community resources available in the areas of recreation, music, entertainment, supplies and so forth.

Counsels personnel regarding safety measures necessary in all patient activities.

Counsels personnel regarding contraindicated O.T. materials and equipment which are available to patients.

Assists in the recruitment of volunteers.

Develops and supervises a training program for volunteers assigned to the activity program.

Assists in any other way to uphold the philosophy of rehabilitation, the objectives of occupational therapy, the work of the activity supervisor and the welfare of the patients.

AGREEMENT FOR OCCUPATIONAL THERAPY SERVICES

I. *Purpose:*
The purpose of this agreement is to arrange for occupational therapy consultation for the *(name of facility)* and to provide for direct occupational therapy services upon written referral by a physician to any patient served by the above facility.

II. *Occupational Therapy Qualifications:*
An occupational therapist (O.T.R.) is currently registered by the American Occupational Therapy Association.

III. *Statement of Functions:*
A. Consultation
   1. The occupational therapist provides consultation to administration regarding program planning, policy development and priority setting regarding occupational therapy service.
   2. Provides consultation to allied professional service workers regarding occupational therapy which includes case finding and case review.
   3. Provides inservice education to the staff of the facility, i.e.:
      a. philosophy and role of occupational therapy
      b. general restorative techniques
      c. physiological and psychological reaction to activity
   4. Maintains a summary of consultation activities in the facility.
B. Direct Service
   1. The occupational therapist provides treatment to any patient in the facility in accordance with physician's orders.
   2. Instructs members of the facility's staff concerning the patient's maintenance program.
   3. Maintains records and reports in accordance with the policies of the facility.
C. Supervision
   1. Provides clinical supervision to other health team personnel, i.e.: certified occupational therapy assistants and activity directors, in accordance with accepted professional practices.

IV. *Responsibilities of:*
A. Occupational Therapist:
   1. Provides services outlined above.
B. Facility:
   1. Provides suitable space and equipment.
   2. Provides services of an activities director to meet the suggested standards of the Department of Public Health, Division of Nursing Homes and Related Facilities.
   3. Cooperates in arranging for consultation and direct service.
   4. Makes available case records and provides for recording services for the occupational therapist.
   5. Provides general orientation for the therapist to facility as well as its policies, recording systems, etc.
C. Mutual:
   1. Provide periodic review of the occupational therapy program, policies, and future considerations.

V. *Terms of Agreement:*
A. The facility agrees to pay the occupational therapist at the rate of $_____ per hour for (number) hours of consultation per month.
B. Direct service will be reimbursed over and above the hours of consultation at the rate of $_____ per treatment.

VI. *Termination of Agreement:*
Should either party wish to terminate the foregoing agreement, thirty days written notice must be given to the other party.

_____O.T.R.

_____Administrator

_____Date

OCCUPATIONAL THERAPY TREATMENT PLANNING OUTLINE
(Use this as a work sheet and attach other pages as necessary.)

Patient's Name_____ First Treat. Date:_____

Room:_____ Age:_____ Sex:_____ Physician:_____

Diagnosis:_____ Date of Onset:_____

Special Problems:_____ Precautions:_____

Adapted Equipment Necessary (Wheelchair, splints, etc.):

Neuromuscular factors:

Passive and active range of motion:

Sensory factors:

Functional status level:

Psychosocial factors:

Other pertinent data:

- -

O.T. GOALS: Referring physician:

Team Evaluation:

Individual therapist:

Patient:

TREATMENT PLAN: Be specific about activities, position, equipment, etc.

SPEECH THERAPY

Speech therapy must be given or supervised by a therapist who meets one of the following requirements: has been granted a certificate of clinical competence in the appropriate area by the American Speech and Hearing Association or meets equivalent education requirements and work experience necessary for such certificate, or has completed the academic and practical requirements for certification and is in the process of accumulating the necessary supervised work experience required for certification.

Speech therapy is service in speech pathology or otology and may include cooperation in the evaluation of patients with speech, hearing or language disorders, determination and recommendation of appropriate speech and hearing services and provision of necessary rehabilitative services for patients with such disabilities.

REHABILITATION SERVICES FOR SPEECH, HEARING AND LANGUAGE DISORDERS

The rehabilitation program should include those services necessary to maintain function or improve the patient's ability to carry out the activities of daily living insofar as communication problems are concerned. These services should include consultant services of professionals in speech and hearing disorders and provisions for speech and hearing testing. Results should be a part of the patient's record. A survey of speech, hearing and language characteristics of all patients is essential in determining the actual needs. This survey should include a special examination using uniform procedures as well as development of a therapy program.

Specific recommendations by the speech pathologist and audiologist should be made for each patient. All cases of hearing loss should be referred to the staff physician. The therapist should provide testing equipment. Those patients requiring more extensive audiological diagnosis should be transported to specialists.

Speech Disabilities

Lip reading should be taught to patients who will benefit from this service, and aphasia victims, usually post-stroke patients, should be retrained in the articulation of ideas. Aids to communication such as charts, large picture cards and large printed vocabulary groupings for patients who can understand but cannot make their wants known by speech or writing, as well as the development of a sign system, are necessary. Eosophageal speech training should be employed where the larynx has been removed. Instruction in obtaining increased movement in structures serving speech is necessary in some cases. The speech therapist will also perform other individual treatment as required.

Auditory Disabilities

Installation of amplification devices, such as television and radio head sets and electronic alerting devices, as well as amplification units in pay telephones, will aid patients who are hard of hearing or deaf.

The speech therapist provides help with hearing aids. This includes securing these devices and obtaining cooperation of local hearing aid dealers in servicing them.

Amplification head sets should be supplied for film programs at the facility.

In-service education of the staff by the speech pathologist and audiologist is beneficial to all members of the facility. Coordination of this program with other restorative services and with the program and staff of the facility as a whole is necessary, and is effected by the speech therapist.

CHAPTER EIGHT

PHARMACEUTICALS— DISPENSING PROCEDURES

All medications treatments should be administered to patients on written order of the attending physician only. Those medications available without prescription, such as aspirin, should also be under the authority of the attending physician.

In the event of an accident or injury to a visitor while on the premises, the charge nurse, supervising nurse or director of nurses may provide immediate nursing care and should notify the administration and the administrative physician immediately. The administration of medicines in this case should only be under the authority of a physician.

Narcotics must be administered only under the written order of a physician —for a particular patient, with a particular dosage, for a particular period of time—with all information being properly recorded in the medical record and on a narcotics sheet.

Included in the transferring of shift responsibility between charge nurses should be a specific narcotics check. All data must be approved by both nurses, and any discrepancies must be reported immediately to the director of nurses.

Unused narcotics assigned, under physician's order, to patients who expire, must be certified as "unused" in the patient's chart and narcotics sheet and must be properly reported to the narcotics authority. Unused narcotics remaining from patients discharged will be handled in the same manner.

No medicine or drugs should be released to any patient on discharge except on the written authority of the attending physician.

A system of patient identification must be made prior to dispensing of any medication.

Only registered nurses may order medication from the pharmacy, and medication may be administered to patients only by registered or licensed practical nurses.

A medicine cabinet with a secure lock must be provided on all nursing units. All narcotics and dangerous drugs must be kept in a narcotics locker within the medicine cabinet under double lock system, with the keys at all times in the possession of the nurse in charge of the unit. Medication may never be stored in patients' rooms. The charge nurse, only, should have access to the medicine cabinet. No other nursing or other personnel should be allowed access to the medicine cabinet. Immediately adjacent to the medicine cabinet should be a sink providing hot and cold running water.

Interuse of medication between patients is prohibited. Medications must be used only for patients for whom they are prescribed and dispensed from a registered pharmacy under the authority of a registered pharmacist.

Labels may under no conditions be changed or altered. Medicines should be stored in the original containers in which they were dispensed from the pharmacy. All medication containers should be labeled with the patient's full name, the physician's name, the prescription number, the name and indicated description of the medicine or drug, the date of issue and date of expiration and, in case of a drug being dispensed from an outside pharmacy, should also contain the name, address and telephone number of the pharmacist and pharmacy issuing the drug. The manufacturer's name and lot or control number of the medication should appear on the label in accordance with the conditions of the Department of Health, Education and Welfare.

Medicines and drugs should be regularly and carefully checked for expiration dates and never used beyond the date of expiration. Upon the date of expiration, they should be removed from the medicine cabinet and either returned to the pharmacy or destroyed under proper authority of the director of nurses and the administration.

Prescriptions should never be renewed unless under the direct authority of the attending physician.

Medicines and drugs requiring refrigeration should be stored in a biological refrigerator adjacent to the medicine cabinet or the nurses' station.

No medication may be ordered for more than thirty days. Narcotics must be reordered after 48 hours. Antibiotics must be reordered after five days. Medicines and drugs ordered for patients suffering from heart diseases must be reordered every fifteen days. P.r.n. medications must be reordered after 15 days. Other stop orders are as follows:

Antianemia drugs	1 month
Antiemetics	3 days
Antihistamines	5 days
Antineoplastics	1 week
Barbiturates	1 month
Cathartics	1 month
Cold preparations	3 days
Cough preparations	5 days
Dermatologicals	1 week
Diuretics	2 weeks
Hormones	1 week
Hypnotics	1 month
Psychotherapeutic agents	1 month
Spasmolytics	2 weeks
Sulfonamides	5 days
Vitamins	1 month

The emergency medication kit(s) will include the following drugs:

Crystodigin
Adrenalin Chloride Solution
Caffeine Sodium Benzoate
Dextrose
Benadryl
Aminophylline
Alidase
Coramine 25%
Levophed
Solu-Cortef

When the seal is broken on the emergency tray, the whole kit must be returned to the pharmacy for re-supply of used drugs.

The facility never dispenses medication for sale. Medications may be dispensed from the emergency tray, by physician's order, in an emergency.

All medications will be properly charted on the patient's chart by the nurse giving the medication. All medication errors and reactions must be immediately reported to the director of nurses, who notifies the patient's physician. In addition, an accident sheet must be accurately and completely filled out and will become a part of the patient's chart. The medication error must also be recorded in the nurses' notes.

TABLE 8–1. PHARMACY DEPARTMENT EMERGENCY DRUG TRAY

Medications			Equipment
Adrenalin Chloride			
Solution (1:1000)	1 cc.	4 ampules	1 airway medium oral
Aminophylline (IV) 250 mgs.	10 cc.	2 ampules	4 alcohol sponges (pre-wrapped)
Amyl Nitrate Perles	0.3 cc.	2 perles	2 files
Aramine Bitartrate 10 mg./cc.	10 cc.	1 vial	1 knife blade and knife handle (disposable)
Atropine Sulfate 0.4 mg./cc.	20 cc.	1 vial	1 #18 gauge needle — 1½"
Calcium Gluconate	10 cc.	1 ampule	1 #18 gauge needle, angiocath
Cedilanid-D 0.2 mg./cc.	4 cc.	1 ampule	2 #21 gauge needles — 1¼"
Coramine 250 mg./cc.	5 cc.	2 ampules	1 #21 gauge needle, Scalpvein
Dextrose 50%	50 cc.	1 ampule	2 #20 gauge needles — 3" intracardiac
Isuprel 1:5000	5 cc.	1 ampule	1 Resusitube
Levophed Bitartrate	4 cc.	2 ampules	1 50 cc. syringe (disposable)
Lorfan Tartrate 1 mg./cc.	10 cc.	1 vial	1 30 cc. syringe (disposable)
Magnesium Sulfate 10%	20 cc.	1 ampule	2 25 cc. syringes with #25 gauge needles
Neo-Synephrine HCl 10 mg./cc.	1 cc.	4 ampules	Attached (disposable)
Pronestyl HCl 100 mg./cc.	10 cc.	1 vial	1 tongue blade, padded (disposable)
Quinidine Gluconate 80 mg./cc.	10 cc.	1 vial	1 tourniquet
Sodium Bicarbonate 3.75 Gm.	50 cc.	1 ampule	
Water for Parenterals	30 cc.	1 vial	

1. The emergency drug kit should be prepared, packaged and sealed by the pharmacist. The kit should be arranged in a manner which permits visibility of each product for ease of selection. Commercial emergency drug kits may be purchased or a fishing tackle box could be used and fitted with a snap-open lock.
2. The kit should contain a list of its contents on the outside cover and within the box. A charge requisition should be included to facilitate patient billing.
3. The kit should be distributed to all nursing stations and other patient care areas.
4. Each kit should be sealed with an easy-open seal to assure availability of drugs when needed.
5. After a kit has been opened it should be returned to the pharmacist and exchanged for a sealed kit. The pharmacist should assume responsibility for the filling and sealing of all emergency drug kits.

CONSULTANT PHARMACIST—POSITION SUMMARY

The consultant pharmacist should be fully responsible for the level and description of inventory within the pharmacy and responsible for the supervision of the preparation and dispensing of all medicines and drugs from the pharmacy to the nurses' station. The consultant pharmacist must be a member of the pharmacy and therapeutics committee of the facility and should function as the secretary of the committee. It is his responsibility to review all medications procedures. It is also his responsibility to implement the policies and procedures as outlined by the pharmacy and therapeutics committee regarding the formulary and in compliance with the *Physician's Desk Reference*. The consultant pharmacist should be available for consultation with the administration, the administrative physician and the director of nurses.

QUALIFICATIONS

The consultant pharmacist must hold a bachelor of science degree in pharmacy.

He must be licensed to practice pharmacy in the state.

He should be a member of the local pharmacy association.

Should preferably have had one or more years of experience as pharmacist in a medical institution.

DUTIES

Supervise the preparation and dispensing of all medicines and drugs, both those brought into the facility and those delivered to the nurses' stations.

Supervise the organization and administration of the medicine cabinet in the nurses' station.

Withdraw obsolete drugs for return, update outdated drugs and medicines.

Provide in-service consultation to charge nurses in the use of medicines and drugs and their applications to patients.

Supervise the operation of the pharmacy.

Participate in the purchasing of drugs and medicines in cooperation with the administration.

Supervise the pharmacy personnel.

Assume responsibility for cleanliness and orderliness of the pharmacy as to the physical plant, equipment, materials and storage of medicines and drugs.

CHAPTER NINE

DIAGNOSTIC, DENTAL AND PODIATRIC SERVICES

DIAGNOSTIC SERVICES

The facility must have provisions for obtaining required clinical, laboratory, x-ray and other diagnostic services. These services may be obtained from a physician's office, a laboratory that is part of a hospital approved by the participation in the Health Insurance for the Aged Program or a laboratory which is approved to provide these services as an independent laboratory under the Supplementary Medical Insurance for the Aged Program.

All diagnostic services may be provided only on the request of a physician. The physician must be notified promptly of the test result.

Arrangements must be made for the transportation of patients, if necessary, to and from the source of service.

Simple tests, such as those customarily done by nursing personnel for diabetic patients, may be done in the facility. All reports must be included in the clinical record.

DENTAL SERVICES

The purpose of the dental program at the facility is to provide adequate professional dental care and oral hygiene for all patients and to develop a nursing care plan that will answer the dental and oral needs of each patient. The facility must assist patients to obtain regular and emergency dental care. A dental consultant should provide consultation, participate in in-service education and recommend policies concerning all hygiene, and should be available in case of an emergency.

Nursing personnel must assist the patient to carry out the dentist's recommendations.

Implementation of the Dental Program

Upon admission, the admitting officer will obtain the patient's dentist's name and address and the date of his last visit to his dentist. The nursing department will notify the dentist of the admission diagnosis. If the patient has not been seen by a dentist for a period of one year, the nursing service will make an appointment with the dentist for the patient, who will be transported to the office for a dental examination. In the event the patient cannot travel, the dentist will be requested to come to the facility.

The patient's chart will be taken with the patient to the dentist's office by one of the facility personnel. The dentist will be asked to write orders for the dental and oral care of this patient. These orders will be reflected in the nursing care plan.

The patient will be taken to the dentist or the dentist will call at the facility at least once a year and at other times, when indicated. In the event a dentist is unable to answer a call after three attempts have been made (*note:* The date of each attempt must be entered in the nurses' notes), the staff dentist will be assigned to this patient. No dental care will be given, however, until the attending physician approves of such care and his approval is noted on the chart.

PODIATRIC SERVICES

It is desirable to obtain the services of a podiatrist to develop a podiatric program for the facility in keeping with the patient's needs. The following points are important to consider in setting up such a program.

The needs of the facility should be determined in terms of patient needs.

The availability of community foot-health resources should be explored.

Podiatric services should be available for both advice and treatment to patients.

An educational program in foot-health care should be made available for staff.

The consultant podiatrist should develop policies and procedures compatible with the health programs of the patients.

The podiatrist should coordinate such a program within the institution.

The podiatrist should establish controls for the program as part of the utilization review plan.

The Podiatric Program

The podiatrist should provide his own instruments and utilize existing facilities to perform his services.

Each patient should have an evaluation as soon after admission as possible to outline immediate as well as long-term treatment needs. These treatment needs should be dealt with at the time of examination, and, where feasible, x-rays, laboratory studies and appliances can be obtained to meet the best interests of the patients.

The podiatric procedure includes aspects of screening, evaluation, treatment, consultation and patient and staff instruction. Proper methods should be employed to satisfy the treatment needs of the patients.

CHAPTER TEN

SOCIAL SERVICES

The medically related social needs of the patient must be identified and services provided to meet them in admission of the patient, during his treatment and care in the facility and in planning for his discharge.

During the process of evaluation of the patient's needs for services in an extended care facility, emotional and social factors must be considered in relation to medical and nursing requirements. Immediately following admission there must be an evaluation, based on medical, nursing and social factors, of the probable duration of the patient's need for care. At this time a plan must be formulated and recorded for providing such care.

Where indications are that financial help will be needed, arrangements must be made promptly for referral to an appropriate agency.

Social and emotional factors related to the patient's illness, to his response to treatment and to his adjustment to care in the facility must be recognized and appropriate action must be taken when necessary to obtain case work services to assist in resolving problems in these areas.

Decisions regarding the patient's discharge from the facility must take into account knowledge of the patient's home situation, financial resources, community resources available to assist him and pertinent information related to his medical and nursing requirements.

There must be a designated member of the staff of the facility who will take responsibility when medically related social problems are recognized and who directs actions necessary to solve them. There must be either a full- or part-time social worker employed by the facility, or a person on the staff who is suited by training or experience in related fields, who is knowledgeable of community resources to deal with social problems.

Confidentiality of Social Data

Pertinent social data and information about the personal and family problems related to the patient's illness and care must be made available only to the attending physician, appropriate members of the nursing staff and other key personnel who are directly involved in the patient's care, or to recognized health or welfare agencies.

The staff member responsible for social services must participate in clinical staff conferences at intervals during the patient's stay in the facility and prior to the discharge of the patient, and there must be evidence in the record of such conferences. The staff members and nurses responsible for the patient's care must confer frequently, and there must be evidence of effective working relationships between them.

Records of pertinent social information, and of action taken to meet social needs, must be maintained for each patient. Signed social service summaries must be entered promptly in the patient's clinical record for the benefit of all staff involved in the care of the patient.

SOCIAL WORKER CONSULTANT—POSITION SUMMARY

The social worker consultant plans, drafts and reviews policies for social services. He aids and supports the facility's social worker, giving advice, counsel and training to him. He consults and works with patients referred to him by the facility's social worker. He evaluates certain patients upon the recommendation of the attending physician or the administrative physician. He evaluates nursing care plans as related to social needs of the patient, and notes certain social needs and fulfillment of those needs on the patient's chart.

QUALIFICATIONS

Master's degree and graduate of a school of social work accredited by the Council on Social Work Education.

Interest in working with elderly, long-term and convalescent patients.

DUTIES

Plan, draft, review and implement policies on social services in the facility.

Aid, support, counsel and supervise the activities of the facility's social worker.

Evaluate patients upon the recommendation of the attendant physician or administrative physician.

Note social needs and responses on the nursing care plan and on the patient's chart.

Develop procedures for the evaluation of each patient admitted to the facility.

Develop forms to evaluate and report patients' needs and fulfillment of needs that are medically related to social needs.

Train the facility's social worker.

Work with patients, their families and the staff in making all parties involved adjust better to the patient's stay in the facility or to his discharge from the facility.

Work with social workers of other social agencies that are serving patients in the facility.

Aid in writing of social summaries when a patient is transferred or discharged.

SOCIAL WORKER—POSITION SUMMARY

The chief function of the social worker is to help the patient, staff and family to solve the problems which retard or prevent the patient's social adjustment or any other problem which affects his ability to benefit from his stay in the facility.

The social worker builds relationships with the patient, his family and friends and the staff. The social worker's activities must be determined by the needs of the individual patient.

From time to time he helps in the in-service training program by giving lectures and holding classes on meeting the social needs of the sick and infirm. He teaches the staff how to recognize the problems and needs of patients and helps the patients to take appropriate action in relation to these problems.

The Social Worker assembles social data about the patients and information about personal and family problems and ensures that this information is held confidential and is only revealed to appropriate members of the nursing staff, to the physician, other key personnel who are directly involved in the patient's care or to any recognized health or welfare agencies.

QUALIFICATIONS

Bachelor of arts degree in sociology or psychology.

Two years' work experience under a social worker or psychiatrist or family counselor (may be substituted for the above requirements of education).

Interest in the well-being of individuals who are aged and infirm.

Ability to build relationships with these people, their families and friends.

DUTIES

Interview each patient admitted.

Interview the family and friends of each patient admitted.

Review social history of each patient admitted.

Confer with social workers who have served any patients in the past or are now serving the patients.

Evaluate the social needs of each patient admitted.

Review the nursing care plans and make suggestions for changes in them when appropriate so that the social needs of the patients may be fully met.

Record in the medical records the response of the patient to social service.

Complete a personality evaluation form on any patient he determines should be so studied, report findings to the physician and enter the form into the medical records.

Aid in the in-service training program and instruct all levels of nursing personnel in understanding emotional problems and social needs of the sick and infirm, recognizing the social problems of the patients and the appropriate actions in relation to them.

Accumulate pertinent social data and information about the personal and family problems related to any patient's illness and care.

Prepare social service summaries on each patient.

Attend conferences by the physicians and staff of the facility before admission of the patient and during intervals of the patient's stay in the facility, and record evidence of such conferences in the medical records prior to the discharge of the patient.

Refer patients and families to appropriate community resources concerning financial matters or social needs that the facility does not provide.

Confer with the social worker consultant whenever required, in addition to regularly scheduled meeting once a month.

CHAPTER ELEVEN

PATIENT ACTIVITIES

Activities suited to the needs and interest of the patients must be provided as an important adjunct to the active treatment program and must be aimed at restoration of self-care and resumption of normal activity. The daily life of the person can be more meaningful if there is an effective program of activities at his disposal. This program should take the following factors into consideration.

These patients are not children, but they have sometimes lost interest in activities and must be encouraged to participate.

Patients can learn new skills, but activities must be geared to their pace because they are usually apprehensive about their ability to learn new things.

These patients must be reassured and often taught that recreation is just as respectable and dignified as work.

With continuous stimulating leadership a patient can be kept in the main-stream of acitivity (within his capabilities) and thus the tendency to withdraw and become overly concerned with his own illness and disability is limited.

The patient must maintain an effective degree of self-respect. Nothing en-hances self-respect more positively than the feeling of being useful. Participa-tion in the planning and implementation of the activities program can often provide this kind of gratification for the patient.

Patients are very often lonely, frightened, unhappy and without substantial friendships. Staff members and other patients are often their only source for comfortable interpersonal relationships.

Some patients will be physically or mentally incapable of participating in organized activities. The staff must plan an individual activity program for these patients.

Patients can benefit frequently from involvement with younger people; in the recreation setting the blending of ages has been found to stimulate the patient into increased participation.

GOALS OF A PATIENT ACTIVITY PROGRAM

Consideration and formulation of patient activity program goals should be realistic and within the reach of the resources and staff capabilities. It should be based on the following:

General health needs of all people.

Health and social needs peculiar to these patients.

General attitudes and concepts concerning health services and standards.

The quality or availability of an active program staff or a program planning supervision and presentation.

The attitude, knowledge and capability of other professional staff in the facility to the program of patient activities.

The *goals* appropriate for an activity program are as follows:

To develop an activity program that will be broad enough in appeal and content to give every patient an opportunity to participate.

To develop the abilities of each patient and provide continuous opportunities for self-expression through participation.

To create and maintain the best atmosphere possible for activity that will initiate and sustain the voluntary participation of the patient.

To develop a program that adds to the total treatment services of the facility and inspires the confidence and cooperation of the staff.

To develop a program that in direction and content will minimize the isolation of the patient from community life.

To make the maximum use of community resources both in the home and within the community.

AREAS AND EQUIPMENT VITAL TO ACTIVITY PROGRAM

Areas:
Lounge area
Arts and crafts area
Group activity area
Outdoor recreation area for sunning, reading, table games.
Outdoor recreation area for sports activities, such as horseshoes.
Outdoor grill.
Equipment:
Card tables
Piano
Phonograph
Rhythm band instruments
Radios
Television

Community Resources

The facility may enlist the services of volunteer organizations to assist in the activity program, such as church clubs, civic clubs, fraternal organizations, volunteer bureaus, private industry and youth groups. Organizations sponsoring large, spectator-type activities in the community, such as circuses, stage shows, movies and variety shows, may be available.

City, county or other public agencies sponsor recreation programs that can be shared by patients of the home. Private societies and associations provide recreation programs for specific ill and disabled groups, such as the blind, aged, arthritic and homebound. Private industry or businesses may contribute to the program by offering donations, money for purchasing equipment or use of facilities.

Crafts for the activity program can be developed using simple resources, from the facility itself—scrap yardgoods, tongue depressors, tape, tin cans; the staff—old nylon hose, small tin cans, newspapers, magazines, plastic; the patients and their families—old greeting cards, old nylon hose, ideas, clothing; the community—lumber yards for scrap lumber, shoe and glove manufacturers for scrap leather, fabric retailers for scrap yardgoods, mills for burlap bags and scrap yardgoods, clubs and organizations for donations of equipment or kits; and the local library—craft instruction and design books, referral to people knowledgeable in specific crafts.

Games, too, can be organized using readily available materials:

From the facility—tables, chairs, specific games, prizes such as candy and fruit; the staff—games they no longer use; the patients and their families—games they no longer use, prizes; the community—samples from retailers to be used as prizes, and volunteers; and from a local church—space for religious services, socials, talks by missionary groups. City recreational programs may also provide sports events and band concerts.

A partial listing of further sources and activities follows:

Parks—picnics, fishing, borrowing of equipment.

Museums and Zoos—special exhibits.

Garden clubs—organize patient garden clubs, organize field trips to flower shows.

Planetariums—special monthly programs that patients can attend.

Aquariums—special programs.

Community—fine arts, arts and crafts, automobile, home, and sports shows.

Civic concerts.

Industries—field trips, sub-contracting work.

Libraries—movies, records, literary groups, book reviews, special programs.

Public schools and local colleges—musical and dramatic groups.

Private music and dance schools—recitals.

Community dramatic productions.

Agriculture and home agents—films, programs, crafts resources.

Health experts—discussions of educational subjects with patients.

Volunteer health agencies—service projects.

Historical Societies.

Senior Citizens Clubs.

The following volunteer service activities within the facility may benefit the patients:

Write and read letters for patients.

Assist in the arts and crafts.

Assist with singing groups.

Play piano.

Operate library or library cart.

Operate motion picture projector.

Assist at parties.

Accompany patients on walks.

Shop for patients.

Sew and mend patients' clothing.

Above all, provision must be made for purposeful activities which are suited to the interests and needs of patients. Suitable activities must be provided for patients unable to leave their rooms. Patients who are able and wish to do so should be assisted to attend religious services. Patients' requests for clergy visitation should be honored and space provided for privacy during visits.

Visiting hours should be flexible and should be posted to permit and encourage visiting by friends and relatives.

A variety of supplies and equipment adequate to satisfy the individual interests of patients must be provided, including books and magazines, daily newspapers, games, stationery and the like.

RECREATION DIRECTOR—POSITION SUMMARY

The recreation director should assume full responsibility for all recreational activities of all patients. The director should participate in the planning and budgeting of equipment, materials and supplies for adequate recreation for patients. The director should be responsible for the programs of volunteers at the facility. The director should plan and organize all the recreation programs, including birthday parties, movies and the like, for all patients.

QUALIFICATIONS

Through either education or training, such knowledge as may have been achieved from a degree in education, or thorough experience in recreational activities at a medical institution.

Thorough knowledge of recreational activities for patients.

Should possess the leadership ability necessary to obtain the cooperation of patients in recreational activities.

Knowledge and willingness to work with patients having limited capacities.

Ability to demonstrate considerable judgment and initiative in adapting special programs to suit the needs of patients.

Ability to secure the cooperation and interest of patients in initiating programs and techniques. Familiar with volunteer programs and able to obtain services of volunteers from among individuals and community organizations.

DUTIES

Organize all social activities.

Provide for the public relations and publicity of the organization.

Speak before civic and community groups, such as garden clubs and libraries, regarding the activities of the organization.

Schedule and supervise all activities of recreation for patients.

Direct outside activities, including picnics, trips and other types of outside parties, for patients.

Direct services to patients through use of volunteers in letter reading and writing and errands.

Maintain data on patient contacts, reactions and patient capacity to participate, and record appropriate entries on nurses' progress notes.

Consult with appropriate staff members regarding patients.

Recruit, classify, schedule and train necessary volunteers to assist in activities.

Determine with the aid of department heads and the administrator where services can be used to best advantage.

Hold periodic meetings with volunteers, giving them opportunities to express themselves.

Maintain a cross-reference file of sources, people and organizations contacted for help or availability.

Keep individual volunteer records, including the age, address, telephone number, hours available, interests, abilities, experience and evaluation of performance.

Prepare periodic reports showing progress, success or failure of activities utilized, and show projected plans for the future.

Have friendly visits with the patients and their families to gather news items for the newsletter.

Be responsible for the ordering of supplies through the proper channels, for storage and the care of equipment.

Read widely in the field of recreational and group activities.

Visit other similar institutions for suggestions on programing.

CHAPTER TWELVE

CLINICAL RECORDS

A clinical record must be maintained for each patient admitted in accordance with accepted professional principles.

The facility must maintain a separate clinical record for each patient admitted with all entries kept current, dated and signed.

CONTENT OF RECORDS

The record must include the following items:

Identification and summary sheet, including patient's name, social security number, marital status, age, sex, home address and religion; names, addresses and telephone numbers of referral agencies (including hospitals) from which admitted, personal physician, dentist and next of kin or other responsible person; admitting diagnosis, final diagnosis, condition on discharge and disposition and any other information needed to meet state requirements.

Initial medical evaluation, including medical history, physical examination, diagnosis and estimation of restoration potential.

Authentication of hospital diagnoses in the form of a hospital summary, discharge sheet or report from a physician who attended the patient in the hospital, or a transfer form used under a transfer agreement.

Physicians' orders, including all medicines, treatments, diet, restorative and special medical procedures required for the safety and well-being of the patient.

Physicians' progress notes, describing significant changes in the patient's condition, written at the time of each visit.

Nurses' notes, containing observations made by the nursing personnel.

Medication and treatment record, including all medications, treatments and special procedures performed for the safety and well-being of the patient.

Laboratory and x-ray reports.

Consultation reports.

Dental report.

Social service notes.

Patient care referral report.

RETENTION OF RECORDS

Clinical records of all patients discharged must be completed promptly and filed in accordance with state law (or for a period of five years in the absence of a state statute).

The facility must have policies providing for the retention and safekeeping of patients' clinical records for the required period of time. If the patient is transferred to another health facility, a copy of the patient's clinical record or an abstract thereof must accompany the patient. This abstract may be in the form of a discharge summary.

CONFIDENTIALITY OF RECORDS

All information contained in the clinical record must be treated as confidential and may be disclosed only to authorized personnel.

STAFF RESPONSIBILITY FOR RECORDS

An employee of the facility must be assigned the responsibility for assuring that records are maintained, completed and preserved. This individual must be trained by an accredited person who is skilled in maintenance and preservation of records.

RESPONSIBILITY OF ATTENDING PHYSICIAN

The attending physician is responsible for the quality of medical care given to his patients, and he is also responsible for health record entries for each patient covering such subjects as history, physical examination, diagnosis, orders and progress notes. Each record must contain adequate data to give a complete history of the diagnosis, treatment and end results of the case. Each entry requiring the physician's complete legal signature should be signed in ink. Initials may be used *only* if the physician can be identified by these initials without danger or confusion with another physician.

IDENTIFICATION AND SUMMARY SHEET

The identification and summary sheet contains two parts: the first part of the sheet contains social information regarding the patient, and the second

NURSING HOME RECORD FLOW CHART

PRE-ADMISSION →
1. Transfer or referral form from hospital or physician

2. Social summary or patient questionnaire

ADMISSION →
Identification data
Patient register and number assignment
Health aids, valuables (and clothing?)
Notification to dietary and other departments
Financial agreements
Legal forms (for psychiatric patients, those with guardians; releases from responsibility; releases of information consents to care, transfers to hospital, etc.
Patient index card

NURSING STATION →
Make up record in the following order or to suit needs:*

Orders
Progress notes (Doctors et al.)

Nurses' Progress notes
Medication and treatment; graphs, etc.
Laboratory and X-ray
Dental
Physical therapy
Admitting evaluation (history and physical examination)
Transfer and referral
Identification and summary sheet

(Headings on each sheet should be written in before anything is written on the form.)

*This is not the order of the chart after discharge.

HEALTH RECORD

(All services feed information into the record during the stay of the patient.)

Doctor →
Dentist →
Nurse →
Therapist →
Laboratory and X-ray →
Consultant →
Dietitian →

NURSING HOME RECORD FLOW CHART (Continued)

DISCHARGE

(Record is delivered to the person assigned to health records, who does the following)

1. Sort the record as follows or to suit (just be consistent and place all patients' records in the same order):

   Identification and summary sheet
   Transfer or Referral
   Admitting evaluation (history and physical)
   Laboratory and x-ray
   Dental
   Physical therapy
   Progress notes (doctors, dentists, therapists, etc.)

   Orders
   Medications and treatments
   Graphic and special reports (if necessary)
   Nurses' notes
   Consents, releases, legal papers, correspondence, etc.

2. Place each section in chronological order—first date first.
3. Check for missing items, signatures, etc.
4. Remind those who need to complete portions of record.
5. See that deficiencies are completed.
6. Code according to disease, if necessary.
7. File for _____ years in numerical order, preferably, by unit system (patient gets same number on each admission).
8. File patient card in permanent card file (alphabetically).
9. Record discharge according to date, file number, name and diagnosis in register (if this is helpful).
10. Record any statistical information which may be needed by administration, state licensing agency, utilization committee or other individual.
11. If a patient is transferred temporarily to a hospital but is to return in a known period of time and a bed is being held for him, the record may remain open. If a patient is discharged to his own home or hospital with no arrangement to return, then the patient should be officially discharged. If the patient intends to return and does not or dies, then the record should so state and should be closed on the date determined by administration. If return is at all doubtful and a bed is not being held, then give the patient a discharge.
12. Statistics may be as detailed as needed for a particular institution.
13. Nursing care plan: Information is summarized from the patient's record to assist the nurse in a quick appraisal of the case. This may be on a card or a sheet—may even be on the patient's record, but usually it is in a Kardex file.
14. Narcotics record: Keep according to state law—refer to pharmacist.

section of the sheet contains the medical information, including final diagnosis and condition on discharge. The physician is responsible for writing the final diagnosis and condition of the patient at discharge and for signing the form at the bottom. The date and time of discharge as well as the place to which the patient was discharged must be filled in by the individual in charge. An identification and summary sheet form is included in this chapter.

ADMITTING EVALUATION

Not later than 24 hours after the patient is admitted, the physician should write a history of the case. It should include the chief complaint, the histories of the present illness and past illnesses and the family and social history. The chief complaint should be recorded in a concise statement, listing the date it began and how long it has lasted. The past history should list the childhood and adult diseases, operations and injuries, with dates for each. The family history should include descriptions of the health of the parents, brothers, sisters and children of the patient if living and descriptions of the causes of their deaths if deceased. Any familial disease should be noted. The social history should describe the social situation of the patient (where does he live, does he have friends, what is his work, and so forth) and the family interaction (how close is his relationship to his father, mother, brothers, sisters, children). In brief, then, the admitting evaluation performed by the physician should include a complete history of the patient on a special form, a sample of which is included in this chapter.

PHYSICAL EXAMINATION

In addition to the physical examination performed by the physician on admission, a physical examination must be performed by the physician at least annually on long-term patients. This physical examination should include all the items listed in the original examination, indicating significant changes in the patient's condition and any changes in the treatment plan. A reminder file is useful for keeping physicians aware of this examination. This file is simply a card index, organized in sequence by date, which is used to remind the record librarian of the days or months when these examinations should be performed. When the patient is discharged, this reminder file card may be removed and stored in discharged patients record.

QUANTITATIVE REVIEW

Within 72 hours after admission of a patient, a quantitative review of the record should be made in order to determine that all parts of the record are included. An admitting check-off list can be used in the review and should list all of the items which should be finished within the first 48 hours of admission. In order to assure that any omitted information is included, a reminder form may be completed and forwarded to those individuals responsible for supplying the indicated information.

PHYSICIAN'S ORDERS

The physician must write and sign orders covering medication, tests, treatments and diets. All orders should include the date on which they are written and the full signature of the physician. A physician's order given orally should be recorded and must be signed by the physician no later than 72 hours following the verbal order. It is preferable that these verbal orders be signed by the physician within 24 hours. Orders must be reviewed by the physician at least every 30 days. Drugs must be ordered for a specific length of time by the physician, and this time must be written as part of the order. It should be understood that automatic stop orders on dangerous medications are a routine procedure and will go into effect in all cases.

AUTOMATIC STOP ORDERS

All medications such as narcotics, sedatives, stimulants, antibiotics, tranquilizers and anticoagulants must be discontinued after seven days unless ordered specifically for a longer time by the attending physician. When the stop order goes into effect, the physician must be notified that the drugs are being discontinued. No prescription should be refilled or reordered without the written authorization of the attending physician. A physician's orders form is included in this chapter.

Devices that are restrictive and considered restraints should be used primarily for the benefit of the patient in his treatment program and should require written medical prescription. Stop orders on restraints should be a routine procedure and must apply in all cases. An automatic stop system must be provided so that any device of a restrictive nature may be discontinued after a limited period of time and cannot be re-employed without a written prescription by the responsible physician.

A discharge order, temporary leave order or temporary transfer order should be written and signed prior to discharge, leave or transfer of the patient.

PROGRESS NOTES

These notes consist of statements about the patient's progress as seen by the individual staff members of the health facility. They include statements about reaction to treatment, general attitudes affecting treatment and notations of change in treatment. These notes should give a chronological picture of the patient during his stay at the facility. They must be written by the physician, and may be written by the dentist, professional nurse, consultants or other professional personnel, each in the field of his own specialty. The writer must date and sign the note he has written and should state his specialty. A progress notes form is included in this chapter.

NURSES' PROGRESS NOTES

It is preferable that the nurses' progress notes be kept on a separate form. These notes should begin with an admitting note showing the general condition of the patient at the time of admission (ambulatory, bedfast, bed sores and so forth). They should end with a discharge note stating the condition of the patient at the time of release from the facility, by what means he left (stretcher, wheel chair, ambulatory) and into whose care he was discharged. The date and time of temporary leave or transfer, as well as the return time and date, should be recorded in the notes by the nurse. The nursing section of the progress notes should be limited to meaningful observations. All notes must be dated and signed by the person making and recording the observations. The reaction to a drug, any apparent change in the condition of the patient and any accident should be recorded. The date and time of these occurrences should be noted and signed. A nurses' progress notes form will be found in this chapter.

MEDICATION AND TREATMENT RECORD

All medicines and treatments should be prepared, administered and recorded on the patient's record by a qualified nurse. After a drug has been discontinued or the patient has been discharged, the remaining portion of the drug should be accounted for on the medical record. A notation should be made in the notes that the medication has been destroyed, given to the patient or returned to the pharmacy.

The nurse giving the medication or treatment must be identified by signature on the sheet in one location, and thereafter initials may be used on a daily basis. A medication and treatment record form is included in this chapter.

SPECIAL FORMS

A temperature, pulse and respiration sheet is to be included in the record. A suggested form is included in this chapter. A special report form for attaching reports with laboratory, x-ray and other significant information is also included, as well as forms for diabetic tests and records of antibiotics used.

Other reports, such as psychological evaluations and physical therapy, occupational therapy, activity and special reports, should also be filed in the health record. The original record (with the signature of the responsible person) should be in the permanent record. Forms containing other information that does not fall under the headings listed previously should be filed at the end of the record when the patient is discharged. Such forms may include legal papers, admission financial agreements, consent to care forms, health aids and valuables list, power of attorney papers and so forth.

RELEASES

A release from responsibility for leave of absence should be signed by the patient or the person legally responsible for him when he leaves the facility for a short time and expects to return. A release from responsibility for discharge should be signed by the patient or his responsible agent when the patient wishes to leave against the doctor's advice. Consent for autopsy should be signed by the nearest of kin.

Each day a review of the records of those patients who were discharged in some fashion the preceding day should be made in order that any missing data can be supplied and errors corrected.

NARCOTIC RECORD—RULES AND REGULATIONS

There must be a separate narcotics cabinet locked within the medicine cabinet, which is also locked. Stored in this cabinet should be all narcotics, barbiturates, amphetamines and other dangerous drugs. An individual "Patient's narcotic record" must be kept and completed for each drug, with an entry made each time one is prescribed for each patient. Accompanying this narcotic record should be a doctor's order for each narcotic ordered for each patient. The narcotic sheet should be completed as follows:

Patient Name — Patient's full name, last name followed by first name and middle initial.

Date of Admission — Date patient was admitted to the facility.

Physician — The full name and telephone number of the physician prescribing the narcotic.

Medication — Full description of the narcotic must be entered exactly as ordered by the doctor in the doctor's order sheet.

Dosage — The exact dosage ordered by the doctor, including the form of the drug used, must be recorded.

Administration — The exact method by which the drug is administered must be recorded, such as intramuscularly, orally or other.

Quantity — The record should show the exact amount ordered from the pharmacy.

Received — The number of units of the narcotic received from the pharmacy must be recorded.

Prescription Number — The pharmacy prescription number must be recorded.

Pharmacist's Name — The full name of the pharmacist dispensing the narcotic must be recorded.

Nurse — The full signature of the licensed or registered nurse giving the narcotic to the patient must be recorded.

Date — The full date by day, month and year wherein the drug is administered must be recorded.

Time — The exact hour of day or night at which the drug is administered must be recorded.

Inventory — After each administration and each recording on the narcotic sheet is made, a balance or inventory of remaining doses must be made on the sheet.

Remaining Doses — After each administration, the number of doses remaining to be given of the drug must be recorded.

Number of Treatments — After each recording, the total number of doses given to the patient must be recorded.

Final Inventory — Each new dispensing from the pharmacy must be recorded and added to the inventories of both the drug and the doses. All columns must balance on each line, so that if the amount on hand shows 60 and five doses are subtracted from the amount on hand, then "5" should be entered in the amount given column and "55" should be entered in the amount remaining column. Should a quantity be received from the pharmacy in the number of "30", then this number should be added to the remaining amount, "55," and the new amount recorded as "85."

Unused Narcotics—In the event that the narcotic is discontinued by the doctor or the patient is discharged, only those narcotics sealed in their original container may be returned to the pharmacy. All remaining unused narcotics must be destroyed before a witness who should be at least a charge nurse, preferably a supervising nurse or the director of nurses. The record should be signed by both personnel and the narcotic sheet entered into the patient's medical record. In those states where unused narcotics must be returned to the proper health authority the procedure described above should be followed, except for the destruction of the narcotic, and the narcotic with the narcotic sheet should be turned over to the proper health authority to be discarded by him.

Narcotic Sheet—*Instructions*—All entries on a narcotic sheet must be made in ink. Each time a drug is administered to a patient a separate line must be completed and a separate entry made. Each new order from the pharmacy must be entered on a new sheet. This sheet should record the inventory transfers from the previous sheet as "unused," the amount received on the new prescription and the total. All patient information must be completed where errors are made—erasures are not allowed. A simple line in ink should be drawn through the error. Narcotics ordered for one patient may not be used for another patient.

Violations of any or all of these rules are subject to prosecution. Note that narcotics recording is probably the most important inventory keeping at the nurses' station that will be done for any procedure.

MEDICATION RECORD—ENTRY INSTRUCTIONS

There are also specific rules that apply to the recording of medications other than narcotics and dangerous drugs. These rules must be complied with and followed precisely. The following entries must be made:

Patient—The full name of the patient must be recorded on the medication sheet, starting with the last name and followed by the first name and middle initial.

Patient Location—The exact identification of the patient, including the patient number and bed number, must be recorded on the medication sheet.

Physician—The full name of the physician ordering the medication, exactly as his name appears on the doctor's order sheet, must be recorded in the medication sheet.

Date—The full date of medication order must be recorded on the medication sheet—the day, the month and the year of the order.

Medication—The licensed practical or registered nurse responsible for the dispensing and administration of the medication to the patient must enter her initials on the medication sheet next to the name of the drug. It is important that the entry in the medicine sheet be accurate and complete. This includes the full name of the drug as ordered by the doctor, the description of the dosage as to the amount and the form used, and the identification of the nursing person administering the drug recorded. Should the same medication be given more than one time in 24 hours, each dosage ordered must be entered exactly the same for each administration.

Treatment—A precise description of the administration of the drug must be given: for example, medicine administered orally to the patient, medication administered subcutaneously to the patient, medicine administered intramuscularly to the patient. The record of each administration must be initialed by the nursing person to show precise identification of the person administering the drug.

Nursing Signature—Each nursing person who has had occasion to administer any medicine or drug to any patient must sign his full name, last name, first name and middle initial, to a section provided on the medication sheet. Following the signature the initials to be used by the nursing person should be written so that they may be compared at a time when necessary. This serves to identify the person who administers the medication to the patient. The exact title of the person should be recorded following the initials, such as "R.N." or "L.P.N." Therefore, an identification such as *Smith, Mary J., R. N.; M. J. S., R. N.* should be recorded on the medication sheet.

ADMITTING CHECK-OFF LIST

NAME OF PATIENT_____

DATE_____

- ☐ Identification data
- ☐ Agreement
- ☐ Health aids
- ☐ Valuables list
- ☐ Transfer or referral form
- ☐ Admitting evaluation
- ☐ Physician's orders
- ☐ Opening nurse's note
- ☐ Temp., Pulse, Respiration
- ☐ Laboratory (if necessary)
- ☐ Dietary notified
- ☐ _____
- ☐ _____

When items have been checked and completed, the list may be destroyed.

REMINDER

To: _____ Date: _____

Name of Patient_____

- ☐ Transfer or referral form
- ☐ Admitting evaluation
- ☐ Orders
- ☐ Progress notes
- ☐ Annual physical examination
- ☐ Referral form to_____
     Hospital or Nursing Home
- ☐ Additional diagnoses
- ☐ Condition on discharge
- ☐ Nurses' notes and reports
- ☐ Signature of physician on Identification and Summary Sheet
- ☐ Signature on _____
- ☐ _____
- ☐ _____
- ☐ _____

DISCHARGE CHECK-OFF LIST

Name of Patient_____

Date_____

- ☐ Final Diagnosis
- ☐ Diagnoses for death certificate
- ☐ Progress notes
- ☐ Referral form to_____
     Hospital or Nursing Home
- ☐ Signature on Identification and Summary Sheet
- ☐ Signature on_____
- ☐ Nurses' notes and reports
- ☐ Business Office notified
- ☐ Dietary notified
- ☐ Release signed, if against medical advice
- ☐ _____
- ☐ _____

When items have been checked and completed, the list may be destroyed.

IDENTIFICATION AND SUMMARY SHEET

To be completed by admitting clerk:

Family Name	First Name			Home phone	File No.

Usual Address			Sex M F	Marital Status M W W D Sep.	Social Security#

Age	Birth Date	Birth Place	Citizen	How long at Usual Address	Military Service Branch Years

Usual Occupation	Kind of Business or Industry	Employer's address and Phone No.

Name of Husband, Wife or Responsible Agent	Address

Name of Father	Maiden Name of Mother

Notify in Case of Emergency	Relationship	Address	Phone No.

Church Affiliation	Name of Clergyman	Address and Phone of Clergyman

Hospital Preference	Insurance

Admitted from	Referred by	Admission Date and Hour

Physician	Address	Phone No.

Dentist	Address	Phone No.

Discharged To	Discharge Date and Hour

Items below to be completed by physician:

FINAL DIAGNOSES:

CONDITION ON DISCHARGE:

_____
Signature of physician

ADMITTING EVALUATION
History

Family Name   File No.

Chief Complaint_____

Present Illness_____
_____
_____

Past History_____
    Childhood
    Diseases_____
    Adult
    Diseases_____
    Operations
    Injuries_____
Family History_____
_____
_____

Social History_____
_____
_____

Inventory by Systems — General_____
    Skin_____
    Head — EENT_____
    Respiratory & Cardiovascular_____

    Gastrointestinal_____
    Genitourinary_____
    Gynecological_____
    Musculoskeletal_____
    Neurological_____
    Psychiatric_____
    Drug Sensitivity_____

ADMITTING EVALUATION
Physical Examination

Family Name _____ First Name _____ File No. _____

General: Age_____ Height_____ Weight_____ BP_____

Communicable Diseases ☐ Yes ☐ No

Skin: _____

Head & Neck: _____

_____

Chest: _____

    Heart: _____

    Lungs: _____

_____

Abdomen: _____

_____

Genitourinary: _____

_____

Musculoskeletal: _____

_____

Neurological: _____

_____

TREATMENT PLAN

_____
_____
_____
_____
_____
_____
_____
_____

Date _____   _____

                                                      Signature of Physician

PROGRESS NOTES

Family Name	First Name	File No.

DATE	EACH NOTE SHOULD BE SIGNED

NURSES' PROGRESS NOTES

Family Name	First Name	File No.

DATE	NURSING CARE NOTES	SIGNATURE

MEDICATION AND TREATMENT RECORD

Family Name		First Name																														File No.	

MEDICATION	Hour Given	1	2	3	4	5	6	7	8	9	10	11	12	13	14	15	16	17	18	19	20	21	22	23	24	25	26	27	28	29	30	31
TREATMENT																																
NURSES' SIGNATURES	SHIFT																															

TEMPERATURE SHEET

Name_____ Case number_____ Ward_____

Date and Ward of admission_____

Month_____ Year_____ Weight (admission)_____ Height_____

Date	1	2	3	4	5	6	7	8	9	10	11	12	13	14	15	16	17	18	19	20	21	22	23	24	25	26	27	28	29	30	31

TEMPERATURE

104
103
102
101
100
99
98
97
96

PULSE

140
130
120
110
100
90
80
70
60

RESPIRATION

50
40
30
20
10

Hemorrhage (grams)	
Sputum (grams)	
Weight	
Blood Pressure	

SPECIAL REPORTS

Family Name	First Name	File No.

URINALYSIS

Name_____Ward_____ Date_____

Physician _____Lab. No. _____

Color_____Character_____ Reaction _____

Specific Gravity_____W.B.C. _____Casts _____

Albumin _____ R.B.C. _____ Bacteria_____

Sugar_____Epith. Cells_____Crystals_____

Acetone_____ Mucus_____Other_____

                                                    Technician

BACTERIOLOGY

Name_____Ward_____ Date_____

Physician _____Lab. No._____

Specimen_____

Gram Stain_____

_____

_____

Culture Report _____

_____

_____   _____Technician

SPECIAL REPORTS — Continued

ANTIBIOTIC SENSITIVITY

Name_____ Ward_____ Date _____

Physician _____ Organism _____ Lab. No._____

Antibiotic	Resis-tant	Sensi-tive	Antibiotic	Resis-tant	Sensi-tive	Antibiotic	Resis-tant	Sensi-tive
Achromycin			Penicillin					
Aureomycin			Streptomycin					
Choromycetin			Terramycin					
Erythromycin			Albamycin					

_____Technician

BLOOD BANK

Name_____ Ward _____ Date _____

Physician_____ Lab. No. _____

Group_____ Rh. Factor_____

Donor_____ Relation_____ Serology_____

Group_____ Rh. Factor_____

Patient's serum & Donor's cells (Major) _____

Patient's cells & Donor's serum (Minor) _____

_____Technician

BLOOD MORPHOLOGY

Hemoglobin ....% RBC .... WBC .... Platelets ....

Prothrombin Time .... Bleeding Time .... Clotting Time .... Reticulocytes ....

Differ-ential:	Myelos.	Juvs.	Stabs	Seg.	Lymph.	Monos.	Eosin.	Baso.	Sed. Rate	1st.hr.	2nd.hr.	Hemato-crit
												v pc

.... Technician

NAME							DIABETIC TEST RECORD					
	URINE TEST		INSULIN		BLOOD	URINE		URINE TEST		INSULIN		BLOOD	URINE
DATE	TIME	SUGAR			SUGAR	ACETONE	DATE	TIME	SUGAR			SUGAR	ACETONE
	B							B					
	D							D					
	S							S					
	HS							HS					
	B							B					
	D							D					
	S							S					
	HS							HS					
	DIET						DIET						

BLOOD MORPHOLOGY

Name .... Ward .... Date ....

Physician .... Lab. No. ....

	Normal Value	Value Found		Normal Value	Value Found		Normal Value	Value Found		Normal Value	Value Found
Glucose	80-120		Tot.Prot.	6.4-8		Ict.Index	2-5		Uric Acid	2-5.6	
B.U.N.	5-28		Albumin	3.8-5		Chlorides*	100-106				
Creatinine	1-2		Globulin	2-2.5		Sodium*	135-147				
Bilirubin	.06-0.8		Ceph.Floc.	0		Calcium*	9-11				
Al.K. Phosph.	0.8-2.3		Thymol Turbidity	0.4-5		Potassium*	3.5-5				
Acid Phosph.	0.13-0.63		Total Cholest.	150-270		SGOT	8-40				
						SGPT	5-33				

* - MEQ/L   ....Technician

RECORD OF ANTIBIOTICS

Name of patient_____ Ward_____

Ordered by_____

Antibiotic	Date started	Dose	Date stopped	Total	Grand total

DEATH REPORT

Name_____ Case No._____ Adm._____

Date of Death_____month_____day 197__at_____M. Unit_____

Age_____years_____months_____days. Was there an Autopsy?_____

Principal cause of death and related causes of importance   Date of Onset

_____   _____

_____   _____

_____   _____

Other contributory causes of importance.   Date of Onset

_____   _____

_____   _____

Symptoms, past week. Pallor_____Cyanosis_____Dyspnea_____Hemorrhage_____

Pain_____Unconscious_____duration_____Edema_____

Date_____197____   Attending Physician_____

PERMIT FOR POST-MORTEM EXAMINATION

Date_____

Permission is hereby given for a post-mortem examination of the
Body_____Brain_____Spinal Cord_____. Check which is to be examined.

Name_____ Patient Number_____

Signed_____

Address_____

Witness_____ Relationship_____

If permission telephoned, indicate here from whom obtained_____

Relationship_____ By whom obtained_____

Clinical diagnosis_____

Other important clinical findings_____

Autopsy performed by_____Date_____

Body to be ready for removal at_____

Remarks_____

INFECTION REPORT

Name _ _ _ _ _ _ _ _ _ _ _ _ _ _ _ _ _

Age _ _ _ _ _ _ _ _ _ Sex _ _ _ _ _ _ _ _

Date of admission _ _ _ _ _ _ _ _ _ _ _ _

Unit _ _ _ _ _ _ _ _ _ Service _ _ _ _ _

1. Was there any evidence of infection at time of admission? Yes ( ) No ( )
2. Did infection develop after admission? Yes ( ) No ( )

> Date infection developed _ _ _ _ _ _ _ _ _ _ _

   A. Type of Infection:

     ☐ Respiratory ☐ Postoperative wound ☐ Urinary ☐ Skin

     ☐ Gastrointestinal ☐ Blood ☐ Eye

     ☐ Other _

   B. Was the infection cultured? ☐ Yes ☐ No

   C. Results of culture _

> (Predominant organism(s)

> Reported by _ _ _ _ _ _ _ _ _ _ _ _ _

> Date _ _ _ _ _ _ _ _ _ _ _ _ _ _ _

Follow-up: (if follow-up surveillance is to be conducted)

3. Date of follow-up _ _ _ _ _ _ _ _ _ _
4. Did infection develop after discharge? _ _ _ _ _ _ Yes _ _ _ _ _ _ No

   (If infection developed after discharge, answer above questions)

> Reported by _ _ _ _ _ _ _ _ _ _ _ _ _

HEALTH RECORD FORMS

SOME RECORD TIPS

There are many companies which design and print record forms, ready for use. These firms will also help you develop forms of logical, easy-to-use design to fit the specific needs of *your* health facility. These companies can advise you about such details as uniformity of size, quality and weight of paper, types of binding and spacing for entries.

It is a good idea in designing forms to bring the physician, the nurse, and the administrative staff together as a team to develop these in a joint effort.

Keep the following tips in mind when developing new forms:

Have only a small supply mimeographed for trial use. Revisions are often necessary.

Keep forms simple and few in number.

Use various colors of paper for quick identification of different forms.

Include at least the name and file number of the patient in the heading. This information may appear at either the top or bottom of the form.

Use standard forms that can be used for more than one purpose. This also helps reduce the bulk.

When possible use a simple method such as a rubber stamp instead of a special form for special entries.

PRINCIPLES OF RECORDING

Be brief! Don't sacrifice necessary facts, but keep records short. Brevity is the essence of effective recording.

All notes should be as brief as is consistent with good communication, and they should have meaning for all members of the staff. Facts should be used rather than opinions.

PROMPT RECORDING FOR CURRENT INFORMATION

By recording promptly all pertinent observations in the patient's record, members of the staff use the most reliable means of regular communication between the physician and themselves.

Each person involved in the patient's care needs to have current information about what others at the facility are doing for him, how the patient is reacting to treatment, what his progress is, and what treatment changes, if any, are recommended.

Use any simple technique for collecting information such as temporary daily assignment cards (the form is included in this section) to check off routine items and significant occurrences while caring for the patient. Information from these cards may then be entered on the patient's health record, and the cards destroyed.

You may find a *nursing care plan card* for each patient (also included in this section) of value in caring for the patient. Items on the card, if written in pencil, may be kept up to date; and later, when the patient is discharged, the charge nurse should destroy the card. The nursing care plan card serves as a worksheet, and it is not part of the permanent health record. These 5 × 8-inch cards may be filed in a visible file at the nursing station. With this filing system the name of the patient on each card may be seen as it is filed horizontally in the small desktop file. If preferred, this information also may be recorded on an 8½ × 11-inch sheet.

RELEASE OF INFORMATION

Information about a patient which is recorded in the health record, as part of the doctor-patient relationship, is confidential. You and your fellow workers in the health care center are responsible for making sure that no unauthorized person *ever* takes any of these records out of the files or reads or copies or otherwise tampers with them in any way at any time, whether it is before, during, or after the patient's stay in your health facility. However, you must remember that some people *are authorized* to get this information, and you should be ready to make it available to them. Because the legal requirements and restrictions about release of medical information vary from state to state, the administration of your facility should ask a local attorney to point out the basic rules to follow.

The attorney should review the regulations of the state administrative agency which is responsible for regulating health facilities (generally, the department of health). Also, the attorney should study the state statutes and judicial decisions about patient medical or health records and tell the staff of your facility what its legal responsibilities are in this concern. He should tell you and the staff what your institution may be liable for if record information is improperly released.

After the lawyer makes this review, your health facility will be able to write a policy about the release of information from health records. This policy will reflect the attitude of *your* particular facility because there are few *specific* laws and regulations concerning health or medical records. Your facility, therefore, must establish within the limits of the law its *own* policies about what information may be released, under what circumstances it may be released and to whom it may be released.

OWNERSHIP OF THE RECORD

The health facility is the owner of the health records. In several states, there are specific regulations stating that the facility is the owner. But even in states where there is no specific regulation or statement, there is no question that as a general proposition the care facility may restrict removal of the record, determine who may see it and decide what kind of information may be copied from it.

Who may see the record? More and more the courts are recognizing the patient's right to have access to the information in his record under reasonable circumstances and for legitimate purposes. In addition, the authorities have gone a step further and extended this recognition to those who are authorized by the patient to see his record and, in some cases, to the patient's spouse. (While the cases in which this recognition has been made dealt with hospitals, there is no reason to assume that a different ruling would be made if a health facility were involved.)

In a few states, statutes give not only the physician and the patient the right to examine and copy the record under certain circumstances, but also an *authorized agent* or spouse. Where these laws exist, of course, the facility must comply.

Although the facility may clearly be the owner of the record, there are some situations in which it cannot exercise absolute control over the release of information from that record. In all states the facility is subject to court orders and subpoenas. A subpoena is an order issued by a court which can direct a witness, such as you or the other members of your staff, to appear and give testimony when the court wants it, where the court wants it and in the way the court wants it.

A *subpoena duces tecum* is a subpoena which also commands that the witness bring and produce certain books, documents, papers and records specified in the subpoena. If you do not obey a subpoena, you can be held in contempt of court.

It should be stressed, in conclusion, that the right of the patient or his duly authorized agent or spouse to have access to his medical records has been upheld by the courts even in the absence of a statute or issuance of a subpoena.

DISCLOSURE OF INFORMATION

The health record usually has at least three distinct parts.

The first part contains information about the patient's identification, such as name, age, address, sex, marital status, date of admission, name of person or agency responsible for the patient, name of referring or attending physician and the like.

The second part of the record contains clinical information about the patient, such as physical examination, history, admitting diagnosis, medication notes, progress notes, nurses' notes, laboratory reports and so forth.

The third part may contain sociological and psychological information about the patient: reports on his attitude, personal likes and dislikes, relationship with his family, behavior characteristics and so forth.

While all the information in the record can be considered confidential, the identification data in the first part of the record is not usually considered as confidential as the data in the second or third parts. Information from any part of the record, however, should be released with care and only when the person requesting it can show a proper and legitimate reason for wanting the information.

In some states, information about the patient which has been acquired in the doctor-patient relationship is considered confidential or "privileged" communication (privileged information may be seen only by certain specified persons). Such information may not be disclosed by the physician in a judicial proceeding unless the patient gives his consent.

Where the law states that the information the doctor obtains from the patient is privileged, a similar status is extended usually, but not always, to the patient's record.

OUTSIDE THE COURTROOM

Rules and statutes concerning confidential information in medical and health records usually do not apply except for court trials or administrative hearings. Other laws or health facility policy will usually tell you whether it is proper to release confidential information in these non-court situations.

Information may be released if it is authorized by the patient or the person duly qualified to represent the patient, such as a guardian, committee or an agency appointed by a court to represent the patient. If you have valid approval from the patient himself or from his properly authorized representative, you will have no problems in releasing information—if you do so exactly as the patient or his representative authorizes.

NOT EVEN THE PATIENT

Strange as it may seem, however, a problem may arise in situations where the patient wants to see his own record. Obviously the patient will consent to a release to himself. The problem is that the information in his record may be detrimental to his well-being. Thus, there is a conflict.

Unless there is some specific legal prohibition in your state about such cases, your health facility may maintain a policy prohibiting patients from seeing their own (or any other) records. This rule, in effect, forces the patient to go to a court and get a court order. On the other hand, your facility may want to impose a rule which is less strict, which allows patients to review all or part of the information in their own records.

WITHOUT THE PATIENT'S CONSENT

Information may be released under certain circumstances without the consent or authorization of the patient.

A court order can force the release.

The health facility may allow physicians and other qualified health personnel to consult its records for purposes of study, statistical evaluation, research and education, insofar as law permits.

Departments and agencies of the government may also consult these records, according to the legal regulations that apply.

Finally your facility may use the records to evaluate its own operations or to protect itself in a law suit.

NOTE: It is imperative for you to remember at all times that if information from a record is disclosed without the consent of the authorized parties, and if it is released for no legitimate purpose, and if the disclosure results in some kind of injury to the patient (being exposed to ridicule, shame, humiliation or suffering is a legal injury), *the patient may have a right to sue the health facility and collect damages.*

The following general principles are suggested for preparing a written policy to cover the release of information to physicians, hospitals, insurance companies, attorneys, government agencies, the press (newspapers, news services, magazines, radio, television, newsreels, free-lance writers, public relations agencies) and others:

1. Requests from doctors, hospitals, social agencies and institutions concerned with the care of a specific patient may be honored only if consistent with legal requirements.

2. Requests from insurance companies and others concerned with the record for commercial or monetary reasons should be honored with consent of the patient concerned. Some insurance policies incorporate the policyholders' authorization for access to medical information as a condition of the insurance, and this provision should ordinarily be honored *unless* there is doubt as to the relevancy of the information requested, *or unless* there is a question of the validity of the proof of authorization. In addition, courts have permitted insurance companies to examine medical records even in the absence of authorization in an insurance policy.

3. An official agency is not entitled to access to records unless it is authorized by law to obtain such information. *Confidential information requested in con-*

nection with security checks for employment or by legislative committees should not be routinely released without the patient's consent.

4. When a court trial or hearing is involved, information should not be released unless the patient has consented. Of course, subpoenas must be obeyed. If a staff doctor or the health facility is a party to the litigation, the affected individuals may have access to the record in order to prepare their case(s).

5. A patient's psychiatric record presents special problems since the patient may not be competent to give permission to others to examine his record. In such cases consent should be obtained from the legal guardian or conservator. It may be desirable to consult the psychiatrist. *When in doubt, however, withhold this type of information.*

6. Be especially careful about releasing information to an employer, even with consent of the patient. It is desirable to give only information directly related to the accident, the disease or the condition for which the employer is paying the cost of treatment and care.

7. *Written authorization* from the patient should be secured before releasing any information to press, radio, television or other news agencies. This kind of disclosure, made contrary to statutory requirements, results in an invasion of the patient's right to privacy AND IS THE AREA OF GREATEST RISK OF LEGAL ACTION AGAINST THE HEALTH FACILITY.

8. When you have any doubt about the release of medical information from the record, get the patient's authorization. The person denied access to the record can always apply for a court order, and this, if issued, relieves the facility —including you— of the responsibility for releasing the information.

ENCOUNTERING CONFLICTS

Refusing to release medical information will sometimes bring the health facility into conflict with the person who wants the information. But if your institution has a consistent, written administrative policy which you apply to each case impartially, the possibilities of conflict and confusion will be slight.

AUTHORIZATION FOR RELEASE OF MEDICAL INFORMATION

Date_____

TO:

You are hereby authorized to release the discharge summary and other pertinent

medical information on _____
                                          NAME OF PATIENT

to the _____

_____
                                          Patient

_____
                          Legal Guarantor or Next of Kin

_____
                          Relationship to Patient

AUTHORIZATION FOR RELEASE OF MEDICAL INFORMATION

DATE _____

TO:

You are hereby authorized to release the discharge summary and other pertinent

medical information on _____
NAME OF PATIENT

to the _____

_____
Admitting/Attending Physician

ARRANGEMENT OF THE HEALTH RECORD

There are no rigid rules you must follow in assembling the complete health record. But you and the staff of your health facility should reach an agreement about how these records are to be put together, and then all records should be assembled in this order.

The order in which the sheets are arranged should meet the needs of your health facility.

When the record becomes bulky, certain sections may be filed elsewhere *if* you are sure that removing them will not hamper treatment or current record needs. Even when removed to another part of the facility, though, they should be kept accessible.

When a patient is discharged, all information concerning his diagnosis, treatment and care should be filed together as a unit. This will constitute his complete health record.

The facility may find it advisable to rearrange the sequence of the health record forms after the patient has been discharged. If your facility wants to follow this practice, you may find that the following order is a workable sequence:

Identification and summary sheet
Transfer or referral statement
Reason for admission and diagnosis
Admission evaluation
Special reports
Progress notes
Orders
Nurses' reports
Miscellaneous

RECORD FILING SYSTEMS AND RETENTION OF RECORDS

The reasons for filing health records are to protect them when they are not in use and to make it easier to find them again—quickly—whenever they are needed.

Your filing system should enable you to identify a patient's record, find that record in the filing system and locate the record when it has been taken out of the filing system. You should make sure that your facility uses the system and methods which do this job best.

Whatever your system, keep the individual record in one place as one unit. A misfiled record is a lost record.

ALPHABETICAL AND NUMERICAL FILING SYSTEMS

The records of patients who have been discharged are filed in either alphabetical order (Adams, Berg, Carlsen, Dupee, etc.) or numerical order (1, 2, 3, 4, etc.).

Alphabetical filing is suitable for a small institution or one having a low patient turnover rate. In this system the record is filed in order by the last name, then first name and middle name, in strict alphabetical order, as follows:

Adams, Abner Hecht
Adams, John Flaherty
Berg, James Alfred
Carlsen, Walter Alex

Two general types of numerical systems are commonly used, the *unit system* and the *serial system*. In larger institutions or in those with short patient stay, numerical filing is recommended. In this system the record is filed by the number assigned, in strict numerical sequence.

In using the numerical filing method a number is assigned at the time of admission. That is, the first patient admitted to your health facility is No. 1, the second is No. 2, and so forth.

If a *unit* system is chosen, a number is assigned in sequence to a given patient when he is first admitted, and each time he is readmitted the same number is assigned to him. For example, Mrs. G. is admitted in March and assigned No. 27 (because she is the 27th patient). She is discharged 5 weeks later. Under the unit system, if Mrs. G. returns to the facility for further treatment, say in November, she would again be assigned No. 27, not a new number. Her patient index card contains the unit number and all dates of admission and discharge. The health record file contains records of all her admissions. If this system is followed, therefore, all records on a given patient will have the same number and will be filed together in one place in the filing system.

In a *serial* system a new number is assigned in sequence to a given patient each time he is admitted. With a serial system, if Mrs. G. came to the facility in March and was the 27th patient admitted, she would be assigned No. 27; but when she returned in November, if she were the 131st patient, she would be assigned No. 131. With this system the records for several admissions of any one patient would be filed in several places. It would be more efficient, however, to file all previous health records of the patient under the latest number assigned, leaving a notation that the record has been moved to the latest number. This is known as the *serial-unit* method and is a variation of serial filing.

During the patient's stay in the facility his record may be kept at the nurses' station or in an area accessible to those making notations on the record but inaccessible to patients and their relatives. It may be kept in a metal holder or some type of individual notebook folder. When the patient is discharged the record should be removed from the metal holder and transferred to the area where it will be stored. There it should be assembled and fastened or placed in a file folder for permanent filing. You should review the record to see that all parts are completed before filing the health record permanently.

Many health facilities file the discharged health record in a file folder because it is easier to file and keep together as a unit. You may select folders made from any of several materials. In some instances, lightweight materials actually wear best, and they also save filing space. Folders with reinforced tops give the most protection because the tops do not crumble and break.

You may store records in letter-type filing cabinets or on shelf files, depending on the size and type of your facility and the amount and location of available space.

RETENTION OF RECORDS

The health record should be kept by your facility as long as required under the statute of limitations or other regulation of the state where your institution is located. The statute of limitations sets a time limit on bringing lawsuits involving patients and their treatment in the health facility. The time limit varies in states and in different types of lawsuits.

In several states, administrative regulations give a specific length of time for keeping all records. In other states, the regulations require that the records be kept permanently.

Where there are no controlling regulations, your administrator, with the advice of an attorney, will want to decide how long your facility should keep its health records for medical and administrative purposes.

INDEXES

Indexes are used to locate information quickly. They give summary information and lead you straight to the health record. Indexes are not necessary unless they are really helpful in the overall functioning of your health record system.

PATIENT INDEX

The patient index is an alphabetical name file of every patient who has ever been admitted to the health facility. It is usually kept in card form (a copy of the form is enclosed in this section) with a separate card for each patient. Many facilities use the patient index, with names listed on 3 × 5-inch cards, as a quick means of finding whether a person is or has been a patient in the facility. Cards are filed alphabetically by the patient's last name, and they list dates of admission and the number(s) assigned to him and his health records.

These cards should be maintained as a perpetual master patient index, particularly if you use a numerical filing system. In a numerical system these cards would be the only source for finding the patient's health record. Basic information for listing on such a card includes the following:

Name of patient
Address
Telephone number
Date of birth
File number
Date of admission
Date of discharge

Additional information, such as whom to contact in case of emergency, may be included to meet the needs of the individual facility. You might include information on diagnosis and complete identification if the card, instead of the full record, is to be kept on file after the statute of limitations or retention period has expired.

The patient index card should be made at the time of the first admission and kept in a file of patients who are currently in the facility. When patients are discharged or die the card can be transferred to the permanent patient index file. The date of discharge or death should be entered on the card before filing. The card should be pulled and used again if the discharged patient is admitted again.

You will need to select a durable and useful type of card for your patient index. When selecting index cards choose those flexible enough for easy insertion into the typewriter yet rigid enough for use in a vertical file. Use standard-size cards for filing in standard filing equipment. The size of the card will depend upon the amount of information you have to record on it.

Since the patient index will expand, the best way to file the cards is in a vertical system with enough guides to make them easy to use.

In vertical filing, cards are placed in a file box or file cabinet, and each card can be read only by pulling the card up. The cards are filed in the patient index alphabetically, by the patient's last name.

PATIENT ADMISSION AND DISCHARGE REGISTER

Many states require that a patient register be kept in a bound volume. If your facility is in such a state you may find it convenient to combine a patient admission and discharge register into a single-bound volume. Information recorded on a register should be kept to the minimum of what is useful to you and what is required by law. It should include only those items which are needed for quick reference and are most easily obtained from this source. The items which might be included in such a combined register are:

Admissions	Discharges
Number	Number (same as assigned at admission)
Name	Name
Date of birth	Date of discharge or death
Date of admission	Discharged (to)
Referral (from)	Diagnosis (including cause of death)

This register may be used to control the assignment of a number to each patient. Each line in the admission column will contain information about one patient, and it will list the number assigned to him. As previously mentioned, in the serial system, including the serial-unit system, the patient is given a consecutive number when he is admitted; that is, the first patient is No. 1, the second is No. 2, the tenth is No. 10 and so on. If discharged and then readmitted at a later date, he is issued a new number, again in sequence. In the unit system the same procedure is used when the patient is admitted for the first time. The difference is that he keeps this same number if readmitted. In the unit system, the number assigned to the patient when he is readmitted is the number on his patient index card.

To avoid confusion in assigning patient numbers, immediately record the name and other information in the admission column when a patient is admitted. This will keep you from assigning the same number to two patients.

USING A DISEASE INDEX

A disease index is a listing of patient records by the disease or condition for which the patient is treated. These diseases or conditions are listed according to the diagnosis given by the physician, and they are listed in uniform terminology. A disease index, however, should be necessary *only* in health facilities where the following conditions are found: first, in a facility which must report its patients by a diagnostic or disease code number to Medical Assistance for the Aged (MAA), Old Age Assistance (OAA) or some other central agency; second, in a facility where research is being conducted.

When a disease index is used, it becomes not only the key to the location of records of patients with certain diseases for purposes of study and research, but it is also useful in compiling certain statistics about medical care given in the facility. And it also gives the facility a good means of counting individuals treated for a certain disease during the year.

A separate card, the form for which is included in this section, is prepared for each of the disease or diagnostic categories. The heading on the card for each disease lists the disease name and its code number. All the cases of the particular disease or diagnosis are recorded on the card for that disease. The data you list on the disease index cards may be simple or detailed, depending on the requirements of your facility. In most instances it may be enough to enter nothing more than the patient's number or name. There are advantages in using patient numbers instead of names, since this saves space and also avoids errors caused when two patients have very similar or identical names.

PROPER NOMENCLATURE

In reporting the diagnosis or disease the physician should use precise and uniform terminology to describe all diseases. For this purpose, the physician should use a nomenclature or system of names of diseases.

Standard Nomenclature of Diseases and Operations, published by Blakiston Division, McGraw-Hill Book Co., New York, is suggested for this use. This nomenclature is familiar to the physician, and he is usually the only one who needs to use it.

STATISTICS

The physician and members of the staff at the health facility, including you, collect the kinds of information needed for making day-to-day decisions, for

PATIENT INDEX CARD

Family Name	First Name	Middle Name	Sex	Age
		Birth date		

Address			Month	Day	Year

Admitted	Discharged	Result	Physician	File No.

(over)

Admitted	Discharged	Result	Physician	File No.

Date	Change of Address

DISEASE INDEX CARD

NUMBER	DISEASE				
File No.	File No.	File No.	File No.	File No.	File No.

making judgments about the service given patients and for furnishing the information required by standard-setting agencies. Much of the information is gathered by reading through the health records of discharged and deceased patients.

These statistics may include total sums or counts of patients and also counts that are combined with others to show such facts as the occupancy, length of stay and death rate of patients. These total figures form the basis for describing the operations of your institution and evaluating the care given the patients.

STANDARD DEFINITIONS

Statistics should be gathered in a uniform way, according to standard definitions. These standard definitions should be agreed upon in advance in order to permit comparisons among nursing homes, for example, and like facilities. There should be a definite reason or use for every bit of material you record, and you should record it in a systematic way. The gathered data should be reviewed at scheduled times so that obsolete material can be discarded and new material added, if necessary.

BASIC DEFINITIONS

The following definitions will be helpful in compiling statistics.

A *patient discharge* is the termination of lodging and the formal release of a patient by the health facility.

The *patient census* is the number of patients occupying beds in the facility at a given time. The census-taking hour is often specified as midnight or any set time during the 24-hour period.

A *patient day* is the unit of measure denoting lodging facilities provided and services rendered to one patient between the census-taking hours on two successive days.

Patient-days of care given during any period consist of the daily totals of the patient census for this period of time.

Discharge patient days are the total number of days each discharge patient had spent in the health facility.

BASIC FORMULAS

The following definitions and formula may be used in the presentation of statistical data.

The *average daily census* is the average number of patients maintained in the facility each day for a given period of time. The average daily census is computed by taking the total number of patient-days of care given throughout the period, divided by the total number of days in that period.

Example: A facility provided a total of 16,425 patient-days of care for the year.

$$\frac{\text{Total number of patient-days of care for that period}}{\text{Total number of days for that period}} \quad \frac{16,425}{365} = \begin{array}{l}\text{45 patients (average}\\\text{daily census)}\end{array}$$

The *percentage of occupancy* is the ratio of actual days to the maximum patient days, as determined by bed capacity, during any given period of time. The percentage of occupancy is computed by dividing the actual number of patient days rendered, by the number of patient days which would have been provided if every bed in the facility had been occupied each day throughout the period.

Example: During the year 16,425 patient-days of care were rendered. The facility maintains 55 beds for patients during the entire year. The maximum number of patient days which would have been provided had every bed been occupied throughout the year would be 365×55 or 20,075.

$$\frac{\text{Total number actual patient-days of care for that period}}{\text{Maximum patient-days of care for that period}} \quad \frac{16,425 \times 100}{20,075} = \begin{matrix} 81.8\% \text{ (per-} \\ \text{centage of} \\ \text{occupancy)} \end{matrix}$$

Average length of stay is the average number of days of service rendered to each patient discharged during a given period. The average length of stay is determined by dividing the total number of patient-days of care rendered to the patients discharged during a given period of time, by the total number of patients who were discharged during that period.

Example: 15,000 patient-days of care were rendered to discharged patients during that period. There were 300 patients discharged during that period.

$$\frac{\text{Total number discharged patient-days of care for that period}}{\text{Total number of patients discharged for that period}} \quad \frac{15,000}{300} = \begin{matrix} 50.0 \text{ days (aver-} \\ \text{age length of stay)} \end{matrix}$$

There are two concepts of *gross death rate:*
a. *Gross death rate* is the ratio of deaths in the nursing facility during any given period of time to the total number of discharges and deaths during that time.

Example: There were 30 deaths during that period. 300 patients (including deaths) were discharged during that period.

$$\frac{\text{Total number of deaths for that period}}{\text{Total number of patients discharged for that period}} \quad \frac{30 \times 100}{300} = \begin{matrix} 10\% \text{ (gross death rate} \\ \text{in a nursing home)} \end{matrix}$$

b. *Gross death rate* is the ratio of deaths in a sheltered home for the aged or geriatric home for the aged, during any given period of time, to the total number of people living in the home during that time.

Example: There were 20 deaths during the period. 150 people (including deaths) were living in the home during the period.

$$\frac{\text{Total number of deaths for that period}}{\text{Total number of people living in the home that period}} \quad \frac{20 \times 100}{150} = \begin{matrix} 13.3\% \text{ (gross death} \\ \text{rate in home for the} \\ \text{aged)} \end{matrix}$$

WHERE DO PATIENTS GO?

All events such as admissions, discharges, temporary hospital transfers, temporary leaves, including absence against medical advice, and deaths should be reported on a daily census report from each section of the facility. Each day that the patient is on a temporary leave, temporary hospital transfer or transfer to a skilled-care unit, his name must appear on the report. This daily census report should also include the number of patients present each day.

From this daily census report, a work sheet should be developed to record these items by number each day. These figures should be tabulated monthly. From these totals the statistical data can be computed. Forms for the daily census report, work sheet and monthly report are included in this section.

DAILY CENSUS REPORT

Section	Date	Time

(A) ADMISSIONS

1. _____
2. _____
3. _____
4. _____
5. _____
6. _____

(B) TEMPORARY TRANSFERS OR REFERRALS TO OTHER FACILITY OR LEAVES--RETURNED

1. _____
2. _____
3. _____
4. _____
5. _____
6. _____

(C) DISCHARGED ALIVE

NO. DAYS STAY

1. _____
2. _____
3. _____
4. _____
5. _____
6. _____

(D) DEATHS

NO. DAYS STAY

1. _____
2. _____
3. _____
4. _____
5. _____
6. _____

(E) TEMPORARY TRANSFERS OR REFERRALS TO OTHER FACILITY OR LEAVES

NAME OF PATIENT	NAME OF FACILITY OR PLACE	EXPECTED RETURN DATE
1.		
2.		
3.		
4.		
5.		
6.		

CENSUS SUMMARY

1. Remaining on last report (line 9) _____
2. Admissions _____
3. Returned from temporary transfers, referrals _____
   to other facility or leaves
4. Subtotal (add 1,2,3) _____
5. Discharged alive _____
6. Deaths _____
7. Temporary transfers, referrals to _____
   other facility or leaves
8. Subtotal (add 5,6,7) _____
9. ACTUAL CENSUS (subtract line _____
   8 from line 4)

DISCHARGE PATIENT DAYS

a. Discharged alive (item 5) _____
b. Deaths (item 6) _____
(F) c. Total discharge patient _____
       days (add a & b)

PATIENT-DAYS OF CARE

a. Actual census (item 9) _____
b. Admitted and discharged _____
   same day
(G) c. Total patient-days of _____
       care (add a & b)

WORK SHEET

Month of _____ **19**_____

| | | FOR   MONTH OF _____ 19___ | | | | | |

DATE	(A) ADMISSIONS	(B) TRANSFER LEAVES RETURNED	(C) DISCHARGED ALIVE	(D) DEATHS	(E) TRANSFERS LEAVES OUTSIDE	(F) DISCHARGED PATIENT DAYS	(G) PATIENT-DAYS OF CARE
1							
2							
3							
4							
5							
6							
7							
8							
9							
10							
11							
12							
13							
14							
15							
16							
17							
18							
19							
20							
21							
22							
23							
24							
25							
26							
27							
28							
29							
30							
31							
TOTALS							

NOTE: Items A through G are taken from the same items on the DAILY CENSUS REPORT

MONTHLY REPORT

Month of_____19___

1. Number of patients present on first day of month _____

2. Admissions _____

3. Temporary transfers, referrals and leaves returned _____

4. Subtotal (add 1, 2, 3) _____

5. Discharged alive _____

6. Deaths _____

7. Temporary transfers, referrals to other facilities or leaves _____

8. Subtotal (add 5, 6, 7) _____

9. Number of patients present on the last day of the month
   (subtract line 8 from line 4) _____

10. Discharge patient days _____

11. Patient-days of care _____

12. Average daily census _____

13. Average length of stay _____

14. Percentage of occupancy _____

15. Gross death rate _____

DEATHS	
NAME	DIAGNOSIS

NURSES' NOTES—CHARTING PROCEDURES

MEDICAL RECORD

The patient's medical record is a complete accounting of the progress of the patient, including the condition on admission, the care and treatment provided and the description of the response of the patient to this course of care.

Complete data must be included to provide for full identification of the patient and all communications with the patient and his family.

A complete history and physical examination of the patient must be recorded at the time of admission, noting past illness, present illness and the plan of care.

Medical Record Contributors

The following professionals and members of service departments all contribute to the medical record of each patient.

Physicians
Nurses
Paramedical personnel
> Physical therapist
> Occupational therapist
> Social service director
> Public health nurse
> X-ray technician
> Laboratory personnel

Consultants in medical specialties
> Dentists
> Podiatrists
> Dietitians

Medical Record Usage

Physician.   The medical record is paramount in importance to the physician in the course of his care and treatment of the patient.

Patient.   The medical record is important to the patient to assure an accurate diagnosis, a proper course of care and a planned program to assure continued health following discharge.

Facility.   The medical record is necessary in order for the facility to properly evaluate its quality of care given and to certify that the care is in fact given in necessary quality and quantity. It is an official record used to determine the financial responsibility for the total care provided to the patient.

Law.   The medical record serves as a legal document in the case of court appearances and litigation concerning the hospitalization of the patient.

Research.   The medical record serves as a document for research to evaluate categorical illnesses and to provide for studies that may result in greater knowledge of medicine and better patient care.

Education.   The medical record serves as a tool to the medical, professional and paramedical specialties for the training of personnel in these fields.

CHARTING REQUIREMENTS

The nurses' notes should contain only significant information in regard to the condition of the patient and his care.

Charting in the nurses' notes should be as specific and objective as possible.

Nurses' charting should include abnormalities observed in the patient as well as normal behavior, changes in vital signs and changes in the social and personal behavior of the patient.

Nurses' charting should avoid all unimportant and, in most cases, meaningless notations that serve only to increase the quantity of the record but may very well decrease the quality.

The administration of narcotics and other dangerous drugs should be specifically recorded in the nurses' notes, and any unusual reactions to these drugs and medicines, as well as other routine treatment, should be recorded.

Every effort should be made to avoid the use of abbreviations and other nonprofessional terminology that may be difficult to understand except to other personnel.

Inasmuch as the medical record is a legal document, erasures of any kind should be avoided and errors corrected by lines drawn through the error with the correction made and explained beneath the error. The charge nurse is responsible for correction of errors in the nurses' section of the medical record.

Notes in the nurses' section of the medical record should be written in ink and should be neat and legible to other nursing personnel and other professional personnel.

The system of color coding in the nurses' section of the medical records should be carried out as recommended by the professional authorities.

Medical Record Information — Nurses' Notes

Observations.   Accurate, definitive and close observation should be made of each patient. Statements of a positive nature should be used in these observations.

Phrases such as "seems to be," "apparently is," "appears to be" and so forth should be avoided.

Recorded Facts.   The nurses' notes should contain the specific complaints of the patient as he has described them.

The nurses' notes should contain observations made by the nursing personnel of physical conditions.

The nurses' notes should contain changes in condition and in the vital signs of the patients, including changes in temperature, pulse, respiration and blood pressure.

The nurses' notes should also contain unusual conditions of the whole patient, including his condition and attitudes, for example, "Patient is stronger (weaker). Patient is bright (lethargic). Patient is depressed (cheerful). Patient is calm (nervous)." In addition, the following factors should be noted.

Patient Color.   Specific notation should be made in regards to changes in the complexion of the patient, such as pallor, flushing, blotching, or signs of cyanosis.

Abdomen.   Observations should be recorded as to changes in the abdomen: distended, hard, soft, painful or tender.

Breath.   Observations of changes in breath odors which might indicate metabolic acidosis or alkalinity should be recorded. Unusual breathing habits (dyspnea) should be recorded.

Temperature.   Changes in patient temperature should be recorded, including outward physical signs of changes in comfort of the patient such as chills or perspiration, along with facts regarding times when these conditions occur. Examples are "Following meals," "During visiting hours," "Certain time of day," "Certain time of night."

Appetite.   Careful attention should be given to the patient's eating habits, including changes in food desires, lack of appetite, nausea and physical and psychological rejection of foods.

Convulsions.   Careful attention should be given to those patients subject to convulsions.

Cough.   Particular care should be exercised in noting the type of cough the patient might be experiencing—harsh or dry, moist, of a wheezing variety or involving expectoration. If the cough is productive a description should accompany the note as to color of the expectorate, its character and thickness.

Delirium.   It is important to note, particularly in aged patients, periods of the day, particularly evening hours and late night hours, when patients might be awakened from sleep with delirium, and whether these patients may easily be aroused from their delirium.

Edema.   Close examination for edema of the extremities should be done regularly.

Eczema.   Rashes should be observed carefully and described precisely in order to determine their etiology.

Eyes, Ears, Nose, Throat.   Regular examinations should be done for abnormalities of the eyes, ears, nose, throat. Eyes should be observed for color, condition of the pupils, irritation or sensitivity and any inflammation, watering, tearing or involuntary movement of the eyeballs.

CONSULTANT MEDICAL RECORD LIBRARIAN— POSITION SUMMARY

The consultant medical record librarian is responsible to act in concert with the administration and the administrative physician to organize and implement a satisfactory form of medical record, including all of the sections important in the recording of the total care to the patient. The consultant librarian is primarily responsible for the review of the medical record on discharge of the patient to determine the completeness of the sections required.

QUALIFICATIONS

Should be registered with the American Society of Registered Medical Record Librarians.

Should have had several years of experience in a medical institution.

Should have experience in supervising a medical records department.

Should have experience in training medical record personnel.

DUTIES

Responsible to organize medical records.

Responsible to advise in the operation of the Medical Records Department.

Responsible to review completion of medical records.

Responsible for training of personnel.

Responsible to be a member of the Medical Records Committee to establish policies and procedures in medical record keeping.

CHAPTER THIRTEEN

TRANSFER AGREEMENTS

The facility must maintain a transfer agreement with one or more hospitals which have entered into agreements with the Secretary of Health, Education and Welfare to participate in the program.

PATIENT TRANSFER

The transfer agreement must provide reasonable assurance that the transfer of patients will be effected between the hospital and the extended care facility whenever such transfer is medically appropriate as determined by the attending physician.

The agreement should be with a hospital close enough to the facility to make the transfer of patients feasible. This transfer agreement shall facilitate continuity of patient care and expedite appropriate care for the patient.

The agreement should be signed by each hospital and the facility to provide for a master agreement and to assure exchanges of information.

INFORMATION INTERCHANGE

The transfer agreement must provide reasonable assurance that there will be interchange of medical and other information necessary or useful in the care and treatment of the individuals transferred between the institutions.

The agreement must establish responsibility for the prompt exchange of patient information to enable each institution to determine whether it can adequately care for the patient and to assure continuity of patient care.

The medical information must include current medical findings, diagnosis, rehabilitation potential, a brief summary of the course of treatment followed in the hospital or facility, nursing and dietary information useful in the care of the patient, ambulation status and pertinent administrative and social information.

167

PATIENT TRANSFER AGREEMENT

THIS AGREEMENT is made as of the _____ day of _____, 19__
by and between _____, a nonprofit corporation (herein
called "Hospital") and _____, (herein called "Nursing Home").

WHEREAS, both the Hospital and Nursing Home desire, by means of this
Agreement, to assist physicians and the parties hereto in the treatment of
patients, (a) by facilitating the timely transfer of patients and medical and
other information necessary or useful in the care and treatment of patients
transferred, (b) in determining whether such patients can be adequately cared
for otherwise than by either of the parties hereto, and (c) to insure continuity of care and treatment appropriate to the needs of the patients in the
Hospital and at the Nursing Home, utilizing the knowledge and other resources
of both facilities in a coordinated and cooperative manner to improve the
professional health care of patients;

NOW, THEREFORE, THIS AGREEMENT WITNESSETH: That in consideration of the
potential advantages accruing to the (a) patients of each of the parties,
(b) their physicians, and (c) the mutual advantages accruing to the parties
hereto, the Hospital and Nursing Home hereby covenant and agree with each
other as follows:

In accordance with the policies and procedures to be established by the
Liaison Committee, as hereinafter provided, upon the recommendation of
an attending physician, who is a member of the medical staff of the Hospital, that such transfer is medically appropriate, such patient shall:

if a patient at the Hospital, be admitted to the Nursing Home, or

if a patient at the Nursing Home, be admitted to the Hospital, as promptly
as possible under the circumstances. Hospital and Nursing Home mutually
agree to exercise their best efforts to provide for prompt admission of
patients provided that all usual, reasonable conditions of admission are
met.

Hospital and Nursing Home agree to provide each other with full and adequate information concerning the other's resources so that either can
determine whether the other can provide the care needed by the patient as
prescribed by his physician.

Hospital and Nursing Home agree:

to arrange for appropriate and safe transportation of the patient,

to arrange for the best possible care of the patient during such transfer,

to transfer the personal effects, including money and valuables, and information relating to the same and be responsible therefor until signed
for by a representative of the party to whom transferred,

that clinical record of a patient transferred shall contain evidence that
the patient was transferred promptly and safely, and

that transfer procedures shall be made known to the patient care personnel
of each of the parties.

PATIENT TRANSFER AGREEMENT — *Continued*

Hospital and Nursing Home agree to transmit with each patient at the time of transfer, or in the case of an emergency, as promptly as possible there-after, an abstract of pertinent medical and other records necessary in order to continue the patient's treatment without interruption and to pro-vide identifying and other information. Such medical and other information must include (a) current medical findings, (b) diagnosis, (c) rehabilitation potential, (d) a brief summary of the course of treatment followed in the hospital or nursing home, (e) nursing and dietary information useful in the care of the patient, and (f) administrative and pertinent social information.

If the services performed by the Hospital are not payable to the Hospital under the terms of any third party insurance or other coverage and, if re-quested by the Nursing Home, the Hospital may bill Nursing Home directly, and Nursing Home assumes responsibility for payment to Hospital, for the reasonable cost of any services, including emergency or outpatient services performed for patients of the Nursing Home. The Hospital assumes respons-ibility for payment to the Nursing Home for services performed solely under identical circumstances.

All other bills incurred with respect to services performed by either Hospital or Nursing Home for patients received from the other pursuant to this Agreement shall be collected by the party rendering such services directly from the patient, third party insurance coverage, or other sources normally billed by the party, and neither Hospital nor Nursing Home shall have any liability to the other for such charges.

Promptly upon the execution hereof, a Liaison Committee shall be formed to facilitate the general implementation of this Agreement. The Liaison Com-mittee shall consist of the Administrators of the Hospital and Nursing Home and such other members as each may designate. The Committee shall have the responsibility to plan and supervise the initial implementation of this Agreement; establish and approve policies and procedures, consider and re-solve problems arising under the Agreement, and recommend revisions thereto, if and as the same become appropriate.

Any dispute which may arise under this Agreement shall first be discussed directly by the Departments of the parties that are directly involved. If the dispute cannot be resolved at this level, it shall be referred to the Liaison Committee for discussion and resolution.

The Board of Directors of the Hospital and the Board of Directors of the Nursing Home shall have exclusive control of the policies, management, assets, and affairs of their respective facilities. Neither party assumes any liability, by virtue of this Agreement, for any debts or other obliga-tions incurred by the other party to this Agreement.

Nothing in this Agreement shall be construed as limiting the right of either to affiliate or contract with any other hospital or nursing home on either a limited or general basis while this Agreement is in effect.

Neither party shall use the name of the other in any promotional or adver-tising material unless review and approval of the intended use shall first be obtained from the party whose name is to be used.

PATIENT TRANSFER AGREEMENT—Continued

This Agreement shall be effective from the date of execution and shall continue in effect indefinitely, except that either party may withdraw by giving sixty (60) days notice in writing to the other party of its intention to withdraw from this Agreement. Withdrawal shall be effective at the expiration of the sixty (60) day notice period. However, if either party shall have its license to operate revoked by the State or become ineligible as a provider of service under Title I. Part I of Public Law 89-97, this Agreement shall terminate on the date such revocation or ineligibility becomes effective.

This Agreement may be modified or amended from time to time by mutual agreement of the parties, and any such modification or amendment shall be attached to and become part of this Agreement.

A confirmed copy of this Agreement with all amendments, if any, together with a copy of the current policies and procedures, referral forms and other documents adopted by the Liaison Committee to implement this Agreement shall be kept in the administrative file of each of the parties for ready reference.

IN WITNESS WHEREOF, the parties hereto have executed this Agreement the day and year first above written.

ATTEST:

_____   By: _____
                                          (for the Hospital)

_____   By: _____
                                          (for the Nursing Home)

The agreement must provide for the transfer of personal effects, particularly money and valuables, and for the transfer of information related to these items.

EXECUTION OF AGREEMENT

The transfer agreement must be in writing and must be signed by individuals authorized to execute such an agreement on behalf of the institutions.

The terms of the transfer agreement must be established jointly by both institutions, and each institution participating in the agreement must maintain a copy of the agreement.

SPECIFICATION OF RESPONSIBILITY

The transfer agreement must specify the responsibilities each institution assumes in the transfer of patients.

The agreement must establish responsibility for notifying the other institution promptly of the impending transfer of a patient. This includes arranging for appropriate and safe transportation and arranging for the care of patients during transfer.

PRESUMED AGREEMENT WHERE NECESSARY FOR PROVISION OF SERVICES

According to HEW regulations, "the facility shall be considered to have a transfer agreement in effect if, and for so long as, it is found that to do so is in the public interest and essential to assuring extended care services for patients in the community eligible for benefits under the following conditions."

In addition, it must be shown "that the facility has exhausted all resources in attempting to arrange a transfer agreement and maintains copies of letters, records of conferences and other evidence to support its claim that it has attempted in good faith to enter into a transfer agreement. All other failures of the hospitals to comply shall presume the approval of transfer agreements."

Requirements for Transfer Agreements under Titles XVIII and XIX of the Social Security Act (Medicare and Medicaid), and by the Joint Commission on Accreditation of Hospitals

PUBLIC LAW 89–97, TITLE XVIII, SECTION 1861 (1), "AGREEMENTS FOR TRANSFER BETWEEN EXTENDED CARE FACILITIES AND HOSPITALS"

"A hospital and an extended care facility shall be considered to have a transfer agreement in effect, if, by reason of a written agreement between them (or in case the two institutions are under common control by reason of a written undertaking by the person or body which controls them) there is reasonable assurance that:

> Transfer of patients will be effected between the hospital and the extended care facility whenever such transfer is medically appropriate as determined by the attending physician; and
>
> there will be interchange of medical and other information necessary or useful in the care and treatment of individuals transferred between the institutions, or in determining whether such individuals can be adequately cared for otherwise than in either of such institutions."

PUBLIC LAW 89–97, TITLE XIX (AS AMENDED BY PUBLIC LAW 90–248, SECTION 234), SECTION 1902 (A) (28) (E)

"A State plan for medical assistance must . . . provide that any skilled nursing home receiving payments under such plan must . . . have arrangements with one or more general hospitals under which such hospital or hospitals will provide needed diagnostic and other services to patients of such nursing homes, and under which such hospital or hospitals agree to timely acceptance, as patients thereof, of acutely ill patients of such nursing home who are in need of hospital care."

JOINT COMMISSION ON ACCREDITATION OF HOSPITALS: STANDARDS FOR ACCREDITATION OF EXTENDED CARE FACILITIES, NURSING CARE FACILITIES, AND RESIDENT CARE FACILITIES. JANUARY 1968. CHAPTER 5, "TRANSFER AGREEMENT"

"The facility has in effect one or more agreements with general hospitals to assure continuity of patient/resident care."

"There shall be a written transfer agreement (reciprocal) with one or more short-term hospitals that shall provide for:

The transfer of patients/residents between the health care facility and the hospital(s) whenever such transfer is medically determined.

The exchange of appropriate medical and administrative information between the facilities."

INDIVIDUAL TRANSFER AGREEMENT

_____ Hospital and _____ Nursing Home believing that the interests of the patient can best be served by assuring continuity of in and post hospital care, hereby agree to the following:

Nothing in this transfer agreement shall be construed as limiting the facility's exclusive control of their separate identity and integrity such as management, assets, debts and other obligations.

Neither institution shall be responsible or assume any responsibility for the moral or legal obligations of the other institution.

The name of neither institution shall be used for any form of publicity or advertising by the other institution without the written consent of the institution of which name is to be used.

Each institution shall have the right to enter into transfer agreements with other institutions.

_____Hospital shall admit patients from _____ Nursing Home upon the request of the patient's physician.

_____ Nursing Home shall retain a bed for the transferred patient and shall accept the patient as soon as the physician discharges the patient from the hospital.

Patients transferred from _____ Nursing Home to _____ Hospital shall be considered on an emergency priority.

Transfer Record Form # _____ shall be completed by the transferring institution and shall accompany the patient to the receiving institution.

The patient shall be held responsible for the inpatient and outpatient charges incurred in each institution. Neither institution shall be responsible for the patient charges.

The patient shall be held responsible for payment of all transferring charges (such as ambulance).

The two institutions shall adopt standardized medical record forms and policies.

Medical records kept in each institution should remain the property of that institution.

The medical staff organization of _____ Hospital shall establish a utilization review committee which shall supervise the medical audit and utilization review of the patients in _____ Nursing Home.

Disputes arising from this transfer agreement shall be resolved by the arbitration committee or persons selected by the two institutions.

INDIVIDUAL TRANSFER AGREEMENT—Continued

This transfer agreement shall be terminated by either institution by notifying the other institution by registered letter sixty (60) days prior to the termination date.

This agreement shall be terminated at once if either of the institutions' licenses to operate is repealed, suspended or placed on probation by any governmental licensing agency.

This transfer agreement shall become effective on _____

_____	_____
Date	Signed Hospital
_____	_____
Date	Signed Hospital
_____	_____
Date	Signed Hospital Medical Staff

COMMUNITY-WIDE TRANSFER AGREEMENT

The hospitals and extended care institutions listed below, all being located in the ___(city)___ area of ___(state)___, do hereby join together in the following community-wide patient transfer agreement in order to provide patient care most suited to the patient's needs. It is the intention of all the parties that this agreement shall operate to promote optimum use of the acute care facilities of general hospitals and of the post-acute care services of extended care institutions.

NOW, THEREFORE, the hospitals and extended care institutions, who are signatories below, in consideration of the mutual advantages occurring to all do hereby covenant and agree each with the other as follows:

The governing body of each hospital signatory below and the governing body of each extended care institution signatory below shall have exclusive control of the management, assets, and affairs of their respective institutions. No party by virtue of this agreement assumes any liability for any debts or obligations of a financial or legal nature incurred by the other parties to this agreement.

No clause of this agreement shall be interpreted as authorizing any signatory institution to look to another signatory institution to pay for services rendered to a patient transferred by virtue of this agreement, except to the extent that such liability would exist separate and apart from this agreement.

When a patient's need for transfer from one signatory institution to another has been determined by the patient's physician, the institution to which transfer is to be made agrees to admit the patient as promptly as possible, provided all conditions of eligibility for admission are met and bed space is available to accommodate that patient, to the extent transfer patients from other signatory institutions.

All signatory institutions agree to set up among themselves standard forms for medical and administrative information to accompany the transferred patient from one signatory institution to another. The medical information shall include, but not be limited to, an abstract of pertinent treatment without interruption. In addition, the parties agree to adopt a standard form to catalog and effect the transfer of a patient's personal effects and valuables.   The intention of this section is to secure for all parties to this agreement the benefits of standardized information and procedures accompanying a patient's transfer between signatory institutions, thus promoting operating efficiency of patient transfers on a community-wide basis.

The signatories to this agreement (shall establish a committee) (agree to use existing councils or associations) to implement, interpret, and coordinate this agreement.

This agreement may be modified and amended from time to time by mutual agreement of all the parties.

COMMUNITY-WIDE TRANSFER AGREEMENT—*Continued*

No signatory institution shall use the name of any other signatory to this community-wide transfer agreement in any promotional or advertising material unless review and approval of the intended use is first obtained from the party whose name is to be used. If information is obtained from the party whose name is to be so used, all signatory parties must agree.

This agreement shall be in force and effect from the time of signing for one year and thereafter from month to month, as long as it is not renounced by any signatory institution by writing to all other parties, giving 90 days notice. In the event any signatory party (or parties) renounces the agreement, the agreement does not constitute an endorsement by any signatory of any other signatory institution, and it shall not be so used.

IN WITNESS WHEREOF the parties hereto have executed this agreement this

_____(day)_____ of _____(year)_____

_____ (institution) _____ (institution)

By _____ (officer) _____ (officer)

_____ (institution) _____ (institution)

By _____ (officer) _____ (officer)

PATIENT TRANSFER FORM

1.

Name	HOSPITAL NO._____
Birth (Last) (First	Transferred Station or
Date_____Sex__S.M.W.D.	From_____Clinic____
Home (Religion)	
Address_____	Address_____
	Date of Date of
Directions_____	Admission_____Transfer_____
Floor___Apt.___Tel._____	Transferred to_____
Responsible Relative or	(Hosp.,Nursing Home,Agency)
Guardian_____	Address_____Claim No.____
(Relation)	Clinic
Address_____Tel._____	Appt._____ Date_____
Physician in Charge	
After Transfer_____	M.D.,City_____

II. Advised of transfer and consent given by   Date_____
                        (Name)   (Religion)

III.

(Check,explain) Impairments Disabilities Mentality ___	Patient knows diagnosis?_____Last Chest X-ray Date____
Amputation ___ Speech ___	Attachments:Diet List__Lab.Report__Exercise Program__Xray Report
Paresis ___ Hearing ___	(Give Dates) IMPORTANT MEDICAL HISTORY AND PROGNOSIS(State
Contracture___ Vision ___	allergies if any)
Decub.Ulcer___ Sensation ___	
Incontinence	
Bowel ___ Bladder ___	

Activity Tolerance Limitations
None__ Moderate__ Severe ___

ORDERS FOR ACTIVE CARE	MAJOR DIAGNOSES
BED	
Position in good body align-	
ment and change position every	
_ _ _ _ _ _.hrs.	PHYSICIAN*S ORDER (Diet, Drugs, etc.)
Avoid_____position.	
Prone position_ _ _times/day	
as tolerated.	
SIT IN CHAIR ____hrs _____times/day	
Increase as tolerated_____.	
SELF CARE	
Maintain__Improve__Level	
Interpret progress to family. _____	
WEIGHT BEARING	
Full__Partial___None_____	
on_____ leg.	
LOCOMOTION	
Walk_____times/day.	
Increase as tolerated_____.	
EXERCISES	
Range of motion___times/day	
to_____	
by patient___nurse_____family.___.	
Other as outlined or attached_____	
Stand ___ Min. _____ times/day.	
SOCIAL ACTIVITIES	
Encourage group _____individual _____	
within _____outside _____ home.	Physician's Sig._____
Transport: Ambulance____Car_____	Date_____
Care for handicapped _____Bus _____	

PATIENT TRANSFER FORM—*Continued*

	Independent	Needs Assistance	Unable to do	IV. PATIENT INFORMATION
				SELF CARE STATUS
				Check level of performance. Use S in column for supervision only. Draw line when item is currently inapplicable.
				In blank space explain assistance needed in care. Use number from table to identify area discussed. Therapists and social workers include title with sig.

	Ind.	Needs	Unable		
Bed Activity				1.Turns	
				2.Sits	
Personal Hygiene				3.Face,Hair,Arms	
				4.Trunk & Perineum	
				5.Lower Extremities	
				6.Bladder Program	
				7.Bowel Program	
Dressing				8.Upper Trunk,Arms	
				9.Lower Trunk,Legs	
				10.Appliance,Splint	
				11.Feeding	
Transfer				12.Sitting	
				13.Standing	
				14.Tub	
				15.Toilet	
Locomotion				16.Wheelchair	
				17.Walking	
				18.Stairs	

19.PERSONAL INTERESTS   Music___
  Group Singing___   Group Games___
  Crafts___ Radio and TV___   Art___
  Plays Instrument___   Other___
20.MENTAL STATUS   Lonely___
  Alert___   Forgetful___ Confused___
  Other___
21.COMMUNICATIONS ABILITY (Yes, No)
  Speaks and Understands   ___
  Writes Intelligibly   ___
  Understands Writing   ___
  (If No or any limitations,describe)
  Responds to Gestures (describe) ___
22.OTHER NURSING INFORMATION
  about diagnosis,medications,treat-
  ments,medical history,habits,pref-
  erences,condition on discharge,etc.
23.EQUIPMENT
  Side Rails Bedboard___Footboard___
  Long:R___ L___ Short:R___ L___
24.BED: Low___ Mattress:Firm___Reg.___
  Other_____

Nurse's Sig._____Tel._____

V.   SOCIAL INFORMATION (Adjustment to disability, emotional support from family, motivation for self care, socializing ability, financial plan, family health problem, etc.)

Agencies Active_____   Sig._____

PATIENT TRANSFER FORM

1. From: _____
   (Referring institution or agency-Name & Address)   (Date)

2. To: _____
   (Receiving institution or agency-Name & Address)

3. _____ 4. _____ 5. _____ 6. _____
   (PATIENT Name-Last, first & initial)   (Birthdate)   (Sex)   (OASI No.)

7. _____ 8. S.M.W. Div. ____ 9. _____
   (Patient's legal residence)   (Circle One)   (Religion)

10. _____ 11. _____
    (Responsible person or agency-Name & Address   (Telephone No.)

12. _____ 13. _____ 14. _____
    (HOSPITAL-Name & Address   (Admission Date)   (Discharge Date)

15. _____ 16. _____ 17. _____
    (E.C.F.-Name & Address   (Admission Date)   (Discharge Date)

18. _____ 19. _____
    (Home Health Agency-Name & Address   (Under supervision from-to)

20. _____ 21. _____
    (Name & Address of attending physician   (Telephone No.)

22. DIAGNOSES
    a) Primary
    b) Secondary

23. Additional Pertinent Medical Information
    a) Prognosis:
    b) Medications:
    c) Treatments and/or therapy   (type):
    d) Chest X-ray   date _____ results _____
       C.B.C.   date _____ results _____
       Serology   date _____ results _____
       Urinalysis   date _____ results _____
       Other laboratory findings _____
       _____
       Other x-ray reports and date _____

    e) Additional laboratory work and/or x-rays scheduled for: _____
                                                              (Date)
       _____
       (Type)

24. _____
    (Signature of person completing this section of report)   (Date)

PATIENT TRANSFER FORM—Continued

(This section to be completed by nursing staff.) please circle as appropriate.

25. Mental Status: a) alert   b) confused   c) forgetful

26. Behavior: a) cooperative   b) belligerent   c) noisy   d) senile
    e) withdrawn   f) socializes

27. Impairments: a) aphasic   b) hearing   c) speech   d) sensation   e) vision
    f) language

28. Incontinence: a) bladder   b) bowel   c) catheter   d) retraining program -
    bowel/bladder

29. Care Status: a) bedridden   b) bed-chair (how long up) _____
    c) amputation (where)_____ d) paralysis (where)_____
    e) contracture (where)_____ f) decubitus ulcer (site)_____

30. Activities of daily living:
    (Please use CODE for items below: I-independent   A-assistance
    U-unable to do)

    a) ambulation   b) transfer   c) dressing

        alone   _____   bed-wheelchair _____   complete   _____
        attendant _____   wheelchair-toilet_____ upper extremities_____
        cane   _____   wheelchair-tub _____   trunk   _____
        walkerette_____   standing   _____   lower extremities_____
        wheelchair_____   sitting   _____   prosthesis _____
        stairs   _____   (type)   _____

    d) hygiene   e) feeding   f) diet

        bathing _____   fork   _____   regular   _____
        dental   _____   spoon _____   blended   _____
        hair   _____   knife _____   liquid   _____
        shaving _____   glass _____   tube fed _____
        toilet   _____   cup   _____   therapeutic _____
                              fed   _____   (type)   _____
                              teaching above _____

    g) weight bearing   h) injections required: yes___ no _____
        full   ____   type _____
        partial ____
        none   ____
        on ___leg

    i) activity limitations: (circle as applies)

        none   bed-rest   moderate   encourage

31. Information regarding day of transfer:

    Bowel movement _____ laxative given _____ if so, time _____ type _____

PATIENT TRANSFER FORM — *Continued*

32. Medication given: _____
                       (include name, strength, dose and time given)

_____

_____

_____

33. Other pertinent information: _____

_____

_____

_____

(Signature of person completing this section of report - phone number and extension)

_____
Date and TIME of report

CHAPTER FOURTEEN

PHYSICAL ENVIRONMENT

SAFETY OF PATIENTS

The facility must be constructed, equipped and maintained to insure the safety of patients and provide a functional, sanitary and comfortable environment.

The facility must comply with all applicable state and local codes governing construction.

Fire resistant and flame-spread ratings of construction materials and finishes must comply with current state and local fire protection codes and ordinances. Permanently attached automatic fire extinguishing systems of adequate capacity must be installed in all areas considered to have special fire hazards, including, but not limited to, boiler rooms, trash rooms and non–fire resistant areas of buildings.

Fire extinguishers must conveniently be located on each floor and in special hazard areas, such as boiler rooms, kitchens, laundries and storage rooms.

Fire regulations must be prominently posted and carefully observed. Doorways, passageways and stair wells must be wide enough for easy evacuation of patients and must be kept free from obstruction at all times. Corridors must be equipped with firmly secured hand rails on each side.

Stair wells, elevators and all vertical shafts with openings must have fire doors kept normally in closed position.

Exit facilities must comply with state and local codes and regulations.

Records of regular inspections by the fire control authority having jurisdiction in the area must be on file in the facility.

The building must be maintained in good repair and kept free of hazards, such as those created by any damaged or defective parts of the building.

FAVORABLE ENVIRONMENT FOR PATIENTS

Lighting levels in all areas of the facility must be adequate. The facility should be free of high brightness, glare and reflecting surfaces that produce discomfort.

Lighting levels must be in accordance with recommendations of the Illuminating Engineering Society.

The use of candles, kerosene, oil lanterns and other open flame methods of illumination is prohibited. There must be an emergency electrical service which covers lights at nursing stations, telephone switchboard, night lights, exit and corridor lights, boiler room and the fire alarm system. If battery operated, the electrical emergency system must be effective for four or more hours.

The heating and air conditioning systems must be capable of maintaining adequate temperatures and providing freedom from drafts.

An adequate supply of hot water for patient use must be available at all times. The temperature of hot water at plumbing fixtures used by patients must be automatically regulated by control valves and should not exceed 110° F.

The facility must be well ventilated through the use of windows, mechanical ventilation or a combination of both.

Rooms in areas which do not have outside windows and which are used by patients or personnel must be provided with functioning mechanical ventilation to change the air on a basis commensurate with the type of occupancy.

All inside bathrooms and toilets must have forced ventilation to the outside. All of these facilities must be located in areas separate from patient units and provided with the necessary washing, drying and ironing equipment.

Installation of elevators and dumbwaiters must comply with all applicable codes.

Elevators must be of sufficient size to accommodate a wheel-stretcher.

NURSING UNIT

The nursing unit must have at least the following basic service areas:
Nurses' station
Medicine storage and preparation area
Space for storage of linen
Equipment and supplies in a utility room
A nurses' call system must register calls at the nurses' station from each patient bed, patient toilet room and each bathtub or shower.
Equipment necessary for charting and record keeping must be provided.
The medication preparation area must be well illuminated and provided with hot and cold running water.

The utility room must be located, designed and equipped so as to provide areas for the separate handling of clean and soiled linen.

Toilet and hand washing facilities must be provided.

PATIENTS' BEDROOMS AND TOILET FACILITIES

Patients' bedrooms must be designed and equipped for adequate nursing care and for the comfort and privacy of patients.

Each bedroom must have or be conveniently located near adequate toilet and bathing facilities.

Each bedroom must have direct access to a corridor and outside exposure with the floor at or above grade level.

Rooms should not have more than four beds with not less than three feet between beds.

In addition to basic patient care equipment each patient unit must have a nurses' call signal, an individual reading light, bedside cabinet, comfortable chair and storage space for clothing and other possessions.

In multiple bedrooms each bed must have flame-proof cubicle curtains or their equivalent.

On floors where wheelchair patients are located there must be at least one toilet room large enough to accommodate wheelchairs.

Each bathtub or shower must be in a separate room or compartment which is large enough to accommodate wheelchair and attendant.

At least one water closet enclosed in a separate room or stall must be provided for each eight beds.

Substantially secured grab bars must be installed in all water closets and bathing fixture compartments.

Doors to patients' bedrooms must never be locked.

FACILITIES FOR ISOLATION

Provision must be made for isolating patients with infectious diseases in well-ventilated single bedrooms having separate toilet and bathing facilities. Such facilities must also be available to provide for the special care of patients who develop acute illnesses while in the facility and of patients in terminal phases of illness.

EXAMINATION ROOM

A special room must be provided for examinations, treatments and other therapeutic procedures.

The room must be of sufficient size and must be equipped with a treatment table, lavatory or sink with other than hand controls, instrument sterilizer, instrument table and necessary instruments and supplies.

There must be areas of sufficient size to accommodate necessary equipment and facilitate the movement of disabled patients. Lavatories and toilets designed for the use of wheelchair patients must be provided in such areas.

DAY ROOM AND DINING AREA

At least one day room or lounge, centrally located, must be provided for diversional and social activities of the patients. In addition, several smaller day rooms convenient to patient bedrooms are desirable.

Dining areas must be large enough to accommodate all patients able to eat out of their rooms. These areas must be well lighted and well ventilated.

TABLE 14–1.   RECOMMENDED VALUES

LOCATION	AREA FIRE RESISTANCE	LIVE LOAD WEIGHT	WALL FINISH	FLOOR FINISH	CEILING HEIGHT AND FINISH	LIGHTING LEVEL
Corridors and interior ramps	1 hour	80 lbs. per sq. ft.	Smooth surface with painted or similar finish. Flame-spread rate less than 25	Smooth water-proof surface, non-slip and wear-resistant	8 ft., acoustically treated. Flame-spread rate less than 25	10 ft. candles
Stairways (other than exits)	2 hours	100 lbs. per sq. ft.	Smooth surface with painted or similar washable surface. Flame-spread rate less than 25	Non-slip and wear-resistant	Equal to wall finish. Flame-spread rate less than 25	20 ft. candles width 3'8"
Exit stairways and landings (Door width 3'8" minimum)	2 hours	100 lbs. per sq. ft.	Smooth surface with painted or similar washable surface. Flame-spread rate less than 25	Non-slip and wear-resistant	Equal to wall finish. Flame-spread rate less than 25	5 ft. candles on floor
Doorways (Width 3'8" [3'10" preferable])	Same as surrounding area		Smooth, durable and waterproof			10 ft. candles
Administrative and lobby areas Appropriate to the size and need of the facility	1 hour	100 lbs. per sq. ft.	Smooth surface with painted or similar finish. Flame-spread rate of less than 25 for lobby and 75 for administrative area	Smooth surface which is wear-resistant	8 ft., acoustically treated. Flame-spread rate same as for wall finish	30 ft. candles
Chapel or quiet area	1 hour	100 lbs. per sq. ft.	Smooth painted or similar finish. Flame-spread rate of less than 25	Smooth surface which is wear-resistant	8 ft., acoustically treated. Flame-spread rate of less than 25	30 ft. candles

Area	Fire resistance	Floor load	Floor finish	Floor surface	Ceiling	Lighting
Physical therapy, occupational therapy and physical activity areas	1 hour	100 lbs. per sq. ft.	Smooth surface with painted or washable finish, waterproof at the base. Flame-spread rate less than 25	Smooth, waterproof surface resistant to heavy wear. *Dry areas*: resilient and slip-resistant. *Wet areas*: Hard tile with slip-resistant surface	8 ft, smooth surface painted with waterproof paint. Flame-spread rate of less than 25	Physical therapy: 20 ft. candles. Occupational therapy: 30 ft. candles
Dining and recreation areas (Combined dining and recreation area should not be less than 25 sq. ft. per bed for 75% of the total number of beds, and should be greater if indicated by the needs of the patients.)	1 hour	100 lbs. per sq. ft.	Smooth surface with painted or similar finish. Flame-spread rate less than 25	Smooth surface which is wear-resistant	8 ft, acoustically treated. Flame-spread rate of less than 25	Dining area: 30 ft. candles Recreation area: 100 ft. candles
Pharmacy area	2 hours	60 lbs. per sq. ft.	Smooth, waterproof, painted, glazed or similar finish. Flame-spread rate of less than 25	Smooth, waterproof finish	8 ft, painted with waterproof paint. Flame-spread rate of less than 25	30 ft. candles. Work table: 100 ft. candles Alcohol vault 10 ft. candles
Patient care unit (Single rooms: 100 sq. ft., preferably 125 sq. ft.) (Multiple rooms: 80 sq. ft., preferably 100 sq. ft.)	1 hour	40 lbs. per sq. ft.	Smooth and easily cleaned. Flame-spread rate of less than 75 in units of not more than 4 patients; more than 4 patients, flame-spread rate should be less than 25	Smooth and easily cleaned	8 ft, smooth and easily cleaned. Flame-spread rate same as for wall finish.	General: 10 ft. candles. Reading: 30 ft. candles

TABLE 14–1.   RECOMMENDED VALUES–Continued

LOCATION	AREA FIRE RESISTANCE	LIVE LOAD WEIGHT	WALL FINISH	FLOOR FINISH	CEILING HEIGHT AND FINISH	LIGHTING LEVEL
Nurses' station	1 hour	40 lbs. per sq. ft.	Smooth and easily cleaned. Flame-spread rate of less than 25	Smooth and easily cleaned	8 ft, smooth and easily cleaned. Flame-spread rate of less than 25	20 ft. candles
Utility rooms	1 hour	60 lbs. per sq. ft.	Waterproof paint or similar glazed finish to a point above splash line. Flame-spread rate of less than 25	Smooth, water-proof and wear-resistant	8 ft, waterproof and acoustically treated. Flame-spread rate of less than 25	20 ft. candles
Kitchen	2 hours	80 lbs. per sq. ft.	Waterproof paint or similar glazed surfaces. The base of the wall should be water-proof and free from spaces which may harbor ants and roaches. Flame-spread rate of less than 25	Waterproof, greaseproof and resistant to heavy wear	10'0", painted with waterproof paint, smooth finish; preferably acoustically treated. Ceiling heights may be lowered if suit-able high capacity exhaust equipment is provided over and above that which is normally required. Flame-spread rate of less than 25	30 ft. candles

Laundry rooms (door widths—4 ft.)	2 hours	150 lbs. per sq. ft.	Smooth, waterproof, painted or similar surface. Flame-spread rate of less than 25	Smooth, waterproof, greaseproof and resistant to heavy wear	Not less than 11'0" except where home-style or small commercial-type laundry equipment is used, and where adequate ventilation is provided. Smooth, waterproof, painted surface. Flame-spread rate of less than 25	30 ft. candles
Janitors' closets	1 hour	60 lbs. per sq. ft.	Smooth waterproof paint or similar glazed finish. The base of the wall should be free from cracks that may harbor insects and rodents. Flame-spread rate of less than 75	Smooth, waterproof, wear-resistant	Not less than 8 ft., waterproof, painted. Flame-spread rate of less than 75	15 ft. candles.
Boiler rooms	2 hours	150 lbs. per sq. ft.	Smooth, waterproof. Flame-spread rate of less than 25	Smooth, waterproof and resistant to heavy wear	Not less than 12 ft., except when domestic-type heating units are installed. Flame-spread rate of less than 25	20 ft. candles

TABLE 14–1. RECOMMENDED VALUES – Continued

LOCATION	AREA FIRE RESISTANCE	LIVE LOAD WEIGHT	WALL FINISH	FLOOR FINISH	CEILING HEIGHT AND FINISH	LIGHTING LEVEL
Toilets (4'5" by 5' with at least one toilet 5'6" on each floor for training purposes)		60 lbs. per sq. ft.	Waterproof, painted, glazed or similar finish. Fire-spread rate of less than 75	Waterproof, wear-resistant and non-slip.	8 ft. (7'6" if lighting fixtures are completely recessed and an approved exhaust system is used for ventilation), waterproof, painted. Flame-spread rate of less than 75	20 ft. candles
Bathing facilities (Shower stall 4' by 4')		60 lbs. per sq. ft.	Waterproof, painted, glazed or similar finish. Fire-spread rate of less than 75	Waterproof, wear-resistant and non-slip	8 ft. (7'6" if lighting fixtures are completely recessed and an approved exhaust system is used for ventilation), waterproof, painted. Flame-spread rate of less than 75	20 ft. candles

TABLE 14–1. RECOMMENDED VALUES – Continued

LOCATION		PASSENGER ELEVATOR	SERVICE ELEVATOR	DUMBWAITER
Elevators and dumbwaiters	Cab size	Not less than 5'4" by 8'0"	Sufficient for stretcher and attendant	24" by 24" by 36"
	Shaft doors	3'10" or larger	3'10" or larger	24 sq. in.
	Load weight capacity	Not less than 3500 lbs.	Not less than 3500 lbs.	Not less than 100 lbs.
	Construction	Metal	Metal	Metal

If a single room is used for dining and diversional and social activities, there must be sufficient space to accommodate all activities and prevent their interference with each other.

KITCHEN OR DIETARY AREAS

Extended care facilities must have a kitchen or dietary area adequate to meet food service needs. It must be arranged and equipped for the refrigeration, storage, preparation and serving of food, as well as for dish and utensil cleaning and refuse storage and removal.

Dietary areas must comply with local health or food handling codes.

Food preparation space must be arranged for the separation of functions and must be located to permit efficient service to patients. This area must not be used for non-dietary functions.

RECOMMENDED LIGHTING LEVELS

Night lights in corridors, toilets, patient rooms and similar areas should yield an illumination of not less than 1 foot-candle. Each bed should have reading light facilities that yield an illumination of at least 30 foot-candles.

The facility must have, in working order, an approved emergency electrical system.

Open-flame methods of illumination should not be used.

AREA	LIGHTING LEVEL (FOOT-CANDLES)
Corridors and interior ramps	10
Stairways other than exits	20
Exit stairways and landings	5 (on floor)
Doorways	10
Administrative and lobby areas	30
Chapel or quiet area	30
Physical therapy	20
Occupational therapy	30
Dining area	30
Recreation area	100
Patient care unit—general	10
Patient care unit—reading	30
Nurses' station	20
Utility rooms	20
Pharmacy area	30
Kitchen	30
Laundry rooms	30
Janitors' closets	15
Boiler rooms	20
Toilet and bathing facilities	20

WATER SUPPLY

The facility must supply, in adequate volume and pressure, water that is free from pathogenic organisms and has desirable physical and chemical properties.

VOLUME AND PRESSURE

The facility will require between 150 and 200 gallons of water per day, per bed. Maximum pressures at fixtures should be a minimum of 15 pounds per square inch and a maximum of 25 pounds per square inch. Approximately 35 gallons of water per minute is required for proper operation of fixtures.

EMERGENCY WATER SUPPLY

An alternate water service or system must be provided. If the facility is connected to a community supply, it is suggested that two service connections or a loop supply be furnished. Where individual water supply is necessary, two separate wells should be provided. Each well should have a pump; these should be driven by internal combustion engines rather than electric motors.

BACTERIAL QUALITY

Source. Water supplies should come from sources that meet the water supply standards of the United States Public Health Service drinking water standards for bacterial and chemical quality.

Testing. The water must be analyzed routinely as a check on its sanitary quality. All state health departments provide such water analysis service. All reports of chemical physical properties of turbidity, color, taste and odor must be kept on file. Water turbidity may not exceed 5, color may not exceed 15 and threshold odor may not exceed 3.

CHEMICAL PROPERTIES

Chemical properties of the water must meet the Public Health Service drinking water standards. There may be some variation from state to state. Your state health department will provide you with data on satisfactory levels through their analysis service.

HARD WATER

Excessively hard water is particularly unsatisfactory for the special uses of the facility. "Hardness" — an excess of 85.5 parts per million of calcium carbonate (5 grains per gallon) — will cause problems in many areas of the facility:

Production of a precipatate with soap suds, leaving film on surfaces of fabric, utensils and instruments.

Increase in the amount of soap required.

Corrosion, encrustation or dissolving of metal from eating away of pipes and other metal surfaces.

Stains on white porcelain fixtures.

Clogging of pipes.

Interference with the operation of some equipment.

Increase in the possibility of back-siphonage in the plumbing system.

WATER SOFTENERS

Should water softeners be used in a facility in an area where water is generally hard, care should be taken in the preparation of salt free diets if a zeolite water softener is used. Care should also be taken when the water supply is high in sodium. The sodium content of the water should be determined by the health department.

The patient's physician or consulting nutritionist should determine whether water softened with such a substance has increased the amount of salt in the diet to such an extent that the permissible sodium level is exceeded. Such soft water may make the salt free diet ineffective.

PLUMBING

The plumbing system of the facility is meant to furnish water to the various parts of the building and to remove liquid wastes and discharge them into the sewer.

The water system must provide sufficient amount of water at proper pressures and temperatures to serve each fixture without allowing back-siphonage of used water to the system.

As previously mentioned, flow pressures of 15 to 25 pounds per square inch and volumes of up to 35 gallons per minute are required.

HOT WATER SUPPLY

Water at different temperatures is required in different fixtures of the facility. The water heating and distribution system must be adequate to supply the following demands:

General use — $4\frac{1}{2}$ gallons per hour per bed at 125° F.

Kitchen use — 4 gallons per hour per bed at 180° F.

Laundry use — $4\frac{1}{2}$ gallons per hour per bed at 180° F.

Hot water storage tanks must have a capacity equal to 80 per cent of the heating capacity. Tanks and heaters must be of an approved type and must be fitted with vacuum and release valves. All water heaters must be thermostatically controlled.

Hot water tanks must be of corrosion-resistant materials.

Burns caused by excessive water temperatures at hand-washing lavatories and bathing facilities must be recorded. Hot water to plumbing fixtures used by patients must be no hotter than 110° F. All bathing facilities in lavatories must be fitted with mixing faucets in order to adjust water temperature. One method of supplying water at different temperatures is to provide hot water at a temperature of 125° F. to all sections of the building and to install booster heaters in locations such as the kitchen and laundry, where water at a higher temperature is required.

Mixing valves may be installed on hot water heaters, thus furnishing water at different temperatures from a single heater.

WASTE SYSTEM

The waste system should provide for quick removal of liquid wastes with minimum chance of stoppage and without allowing vermin or sewer gases to enter the building.

Fixture drain lines, stacks, vents and fixture traps must be of correct size and properly laid out and connected. Local plumbing ordinances and codes regulate these matters. In the absence of local codes the administrator should consult the National Plumbing Code.

Back flow and back siphonage.   Back flow is the flow of water or other liquids into the distribution pipe of a water supply from any source other than its intended source. Back siphonage is the flowing back of used, contaminated or polluted water from a plumbing fixture into a water supply due to a negative pressure in such pipes.

Disease outbreaks have occurred as a result of conditions of back flow or back siphonage. In addition to water supply contamination, back flow and back siphonage may contaminate the interiors of such equipment as autoclaves, instrument boilers and water sterilizers. Back flow of sewage or storm water into basins may also contaminate food, laundry and medical and other supplies, if the basement is flooded.

Vacuum breakers and back flow preventers are devices which will protect fixtures and water supply. They must be installed on the following pieces of equipment:

Flush valves of toilets and urinals.
Bedpan washers and steamers.
Autoclaves and water sterilizer boilers.
Valves of flush rim sinks.
Valves of water flush floor drains.
Aspirators.
Fluid suction systems.
Laboratory sink traps.
Spray hoses.
Dishwashing machines.
Garbage grinders.
Laundry washing machines.
Instrument and equipment boilers.
High speed instrument washers.
Washer sterilizers.
Sterilizers.

Other pieces of specialized equipment which have submerged or submersible water inlets.

Fixed air depths or air breaks must be placed in the waste lines of the following equipment:

Autoclaves.

Instrument and equipment boilers.

Water sterilizers.

High speed instrument washers and sterilizers.

Dishwashing machines.

Walk-in refrigerators.

Potato and vegetable peelers.

Laundry and washing machines.

Laundry extractors.

Other pieces of equipment which discharge into sewer lines in which sewage may back up.

The vents from pressure sterilizing equipment, autoclaves, must be designed and installed to prevent the back flow of condensate into the sterile chamber.

Should frequent flooding of building sewers, building drains or storm sewers occur, back water traps, devices or valves must be installed.

SPECIAL PLUMBING FIXTURES

Special plumbing fixtures have been devised to meet the needs of extended care facilities:

Hand-Washing Lavatory and Controls

Gooseneck faucets must be located on all hand-washing lavatories at nursing stations, examining rooms, utility rooms, kitchens, isolation rooms and similar areas used by nursing and medical staff and food handling personnel. Hand-washing lavatories in patients' rooms should also be fitted with gooseneck faucets.

Hand-washing lavatories with foot-controlled valves should be located at nurses' stations, utility rooms, kitchens, examining rooms and isolation rooms.

Elbow control valves may also be used in place of the foot-controlled valves. Knee-controlled valves may be used in place of foot-controlled valves at lavatory locations as specified above. Wrist- or elbow-operated valves may be used in lieu of foot- or knee-controls. It is recommended that wrist or elbow controls be installed at all patient room lavatories in addition to locations recommended for foot and knee controls.

Bathing Facilities

It is preferable that pear-type bathtubs be installed against walls instead of fitted tubs. These tubs provide working space for nurses on three sides as well as easy access for the patient. Tubs usually are elevated 12 to 16 inches above the floor level.

Showers designed without curbs and with at least one low wall are recommended. Such shower facilities must provide access for wheel chairs and carts. The low wall provides protection to the attendant assisting the patient. The shower should be fitted with spray heads on flexible hoses rather than standard rigid shower heads.

Toilet Fixtures

Each patient room toilet should be fitted with a bedpan cleaning device and bedpan lugs to facilitate the flushing of bed pans and similar equipment.

Flexible hose bedpan flushers must be located on individual patient room toilet fixtures and on clinic service sinks. Flexible hoses should be equipped with foot-operated valves.

Diverter valves are used for flushing bedpans and similar equipment and should be attached to water closets and clinic service sinks with flusher meter valve flushers.

Clinic service sinks are adaptations of the water closet and are used specifically for emptying liquid waste from bedpans and other similar utensils. These fixtures must maintain a water level in the bowl similar to that in a toilet. Such fixtures are located in soiled utility rooms.

Flushing rim sinks are designed for the disposal of liquid wastes only. They are not equipped with strainers and there is no water level in the receptacle. Therefore, solid waste material cannot be carried along with the liquid waste.

The *bedpan flusher–washer combination* is a device that empties, flushes and steams utensils without removing them from the fixture. It is specifically designed for emptying bedpans located in soiled utility rooms. There are obtainable manually operated models or automatically operated models which regulate flushing and steam cycles.

Sterilizing and Disinfecting Equipment

The autoclave.   The autoclave or pressure sterilizer is the only device other than the hot air oven which is used for sterilization of medical supplies. This equipment usually operates at a temperature of 250° F. and 10 to 15 pounds pressure.

Equipment washer—sanitizer.   An adaptation of the dishwasher for medical equipment, this device is used to wash in a fixed cycle and sanitize in the final cycle with free flowing steam.

Boiling sterilizer.   This device is not an actual sterilizer. It is a vessel in which hospital utensils may be placed in racks and immersed in water. The water is heated to boiling temperature but never reaches a temperature above 212° F. Boiling sterilizers are used to clean equipment rather than to actually sterilize.

Deep laundry sink.   The laundry sink may be provided in the utility rooms for disinfection of medical equipment by immersion in chemical solutions.

Bedpan flusher washer.   This device empties, flushes and steams the bedpan by use of water flushing and a steam cycle.

WASTE HANDLING

Improper handling of waste results in attraction of insects and rodents, creates conditions favorable to their propagation and causes offensive odor and unsightly appearance. It also exposes employees to contaminated materials.

Patients of advanced age, and those who are in poor physical condition, are quite vulnerable to infectious diseases. For this reason, as well as those already given, the proper collection, storage and disposal of liquid and solid wastes are essential to maintain the clean environment that is the key to prevention and control of communicable diseases.

INDIVIDUAL LIQUID WASTE DISPOSAL SYSTEMS

All liquid wastes should be discharged into a public sewerage system that is adequate and that has been approved by the proper authorities. If there is no access to such a system, an individual liquid waste disposal system should be constructed on the site of the facility.

A. Design

Individual sewage disposal facilities should be designed by a competent sanitary engineer to meet the needs of the institution.

1. Grease traps

Grease traps should be used on kitchen waste lines if the volume of kitchen wastes is large. They should be readily accessible for cleaning. Accumulated grease should be removed from the trap at regular intervals. This task should be included in the task description and work time schedule.

2. Garbage grinders

Garbage grinders should not be discharged into a grease trap.

3. Laundry wastes

If large quantities of laundry wastes are to be treated in an individual system, a sanitary engineer who is competent in laundry waste treatment should be consulted as to procedure.

B. Maintenance

Maintenance varies with the different types of disposal systems, and its frequency will vary with the adequacy of the system.

1. Responsibility for maintenance

The discharge of this responsibility should be assigned to a specific individual.

2. Training and tools

The individual to whom the responsibility is assigned should be trained in his duties and be provided with proper equipment to carry out his tasks.

3. Systemization

The maintenance activity should be included in a task description manual and a work time schedule.

SOLID WASTE DISPOSAL SYSTEMS

A. Definitions

1. Waste

Waste consists of the useless, used or unwanted materials that result from normal activities, and which are discarded. Wastes can include solids, liquids and gases.

2. Garbage

Garbage is composed of the putrescible animal and vegetable wastes that result from the handling, preparation and consumption of foods.

3. Rubbish

Rubbish consists of all nonputrescible solid wastes except ashes. This includes both combustible and noncombustible materials, such as paper, tin cans, glass bottles, bedding, rags, crockery and metals.

4. Biological wastes

These wastes result directly from patient care, diagnostic procedures and treatment.

5. Refuse

Refuse includes all putrescible and nonputrescible solid wastes, such as garbage, rubbish, ashes and biological wastes.

A *collection system* coordinates administrative and procedural techniques and the use of equipment in the collection, transfer and transport of wastes. An effective *disposal method* is the ultimate means of rendering wastes inoffensive from a public health and public nuisance standpoint.

B. Typical Wastes and Their Origins

1. Patient care activities

Soiled dressings
Bandages
Disposable underpads
Diapers
Catheters
Enema squeeze bottles
Paper tissues soaked with
  body secretions

Sputum receptacles
Masks
Needles and syringes
Swabs
Sanitary napkins
Plaster casts
Paper goods and
  similar items

2. Kitchen and food service area

Metal, glass, plastic and paper containers
Waste food
Discarded utensils
Cloths

3. Nursing stations

Bottles
Ampules
Disposable needles and syringes

Paper goods
Similar items of
metals, glass, plastic or rubber

4. Service areas (laundry, housekeeping, etc.):

Cartons
Crates
Packing materials
Paper goods
Metal containers

Bottles
Vacuum cleaner bags
Rags
Discarded furniture

5. Patient rooms and public areas

Paper goods (including newspapers, magazines)
Flowers
Discarded foods (not from food service)
Bottles

C. Planning Systems to Handle Solid Waste

The system for handling and disposing of solid waste should be planned during the preliminary design phase of the facility. When an existing structure is being remodeled, handling and disposing of solid wastes should be given consideration at an early stage of the planning of changes.

1. Estimating solid waste quantities

There are no adequate data upon which reliable estimates can be based. Approximations may be based on the fact that a 100-bed facility produces about nine pounds of waste per patient per day.

2. Methods of waste disposal

Community collection system.   Community services (public or private), when available, should be used for all solid wastes except infected dressings, surgical dressings and materials that may be contaminated by infectious agents. These latter wastes should be incinerated on the premises.

Incineration of wastes on the premises.   Solid wastes (except metal, glass, and other noncombustibles) can be incinerated without causing a fly or a rodent problem. However, this means of disposal sometimes produces some smoke and odor. If an incinerator is used for all wastes, it should have an auxiliary fuel supply to insure complete combustion of the material. Burning in open drums or fireplaces and similar methods of disposal should never be used in a nursing home.

In some communities special types of incinerators are necessary to meet air pollution control requirements.

Burying.   There must be an adequate area of land available for this purpose, and the wastes should be covered by two feet of earth immediately after being dumped. In general, burial on the premises often proves to be an unsatisfactory means of waste disposal.

Hog feeding (garbage).   This method does not eliminate the need for satisfactory storage and removal of rubbish. Neither is it a complete disposal method. Only the edible garbage is consumed, and both what is left of this portion and the hog manure support insects and rodents. (Also, garbage must be heated to a temperature of 212° F. for at least 30 minutes in most states before being fed to hogs.)

Grinding (garbage).   This method does not eliminate the need for satisfactory storage and removal of rubbish; however, it is an excellent method of garbage disposal. The materials disposed of are reduced to fine particles which discharge in a stream of water into a sanitary sewer or an approved individual sewage disposal system.

3. Estimating equipment capacity

Determine the kinds of waste and the amount of each, and determine the length of time that the wastes must be stored. From these estimations, the number, sizes, types and locations of initial accumulation waste containers can be determined. The same information can be used to determine the size and number of transfer receptacles and transportation vehicles. This information, in conjunction with a knowledge of the frequency of removal of wastes from the premises, can be used to determine the amount of space needed for storage of wastes.

CONTAINERS FOR COLLECTING WASTES WITHIN THE FACILITY

Metal cans.   Thirty-two–gallon galvanized iron cans are suitable for waste from many activities. These cans can be either hand-carried or moved on flatbed trucks to the waste pickup point (if public facilities are used) or to a place of storage or disposal. Metal cans should be washed and disinfected either by chemical agents or with steam.

The advantages of *polyethylene linings for containers* are as follows:

Plastic-lined containers do not have to be washed after each emptying.

Waste-filled plastic liners are less noisy in handling than metal containers.

Depreciation of metal containers is reduced by the use of plastic liners.

All original and transfer containers should be lined with plastic liners. As each container becomes full, remove the liner and included wastes and put the bundle in a transfer container (a closed truck, a galvanized iron can or other equipment).

Maids' carts should have a special bag for the collection of dry wastes. Closed waste carts and bags may be used.

Disposable Single-Service Containers. Special cardboard rubbish containers or single-service draft paper sacks and frame holders can be used for utility areas. About 2.5 cubic feet of rubbish will accumulate in the average utility room each 12 hours. No transfer of rubbish is required when these disposable containers are used because the container as well as the contents can be incinerated. This reduces contact through handling and air contamination. Also, the need to clean and disinfect containers is eliminated, and noise of handling is reduced.

INSECT CONTROL

A. Domestic Flies

These insects transmit enteric diseases to man. Some bite. Fly larvae can infest human flesh and intestines as well as stored foods.

1. Environmental control

Wrap drained garbage and store all refuse in durable cans with tight lids. Maintain insect screening.

2. Chemical control

Indoors: residual spray with 5 per cent DDT; space spray with 0.1 per cent pyrethrum or allethrin. Outdoors: residual spray with 5 per cent Malathion; space spray with 5 per cent DDT or 3 per cent Malathion.

B. Mosquitoes

These insects suck blood and transmit encephalitis and malaria in the United States. Yellow fever and other mosquito-borne diseases could be introduced without warning.

1. Environmental control

Eliminate standing water in cans, tires, rain gutters, catch basins and rain barrels. Also eliminate standing ground surface water.

Maintain insect screening.

2. Chemical control

The control measures listed for flies are effective against mosquitoes.

C. Cockroaches

Cockroaches produce unpleasant odors, nibble on infirm persons, transmit diarrhea and dysentery and damage stored products.

1. Environmental control

Eliminate cracks, crevices and dead spaces. Store food and refuse properly. Keep entire area scrupulously clean. Watch for, and destroy, all cockroaches and their egg cases, particularly those that are introduced with luggage, groceries, furniture and fire wood.

2. Chemical control

Pin-stream spray with insecticides all cracks and crevices, baseboards, furniture, fixtures and cabinets. Use the following:

3 per cent chlordane emulsion.*

1 per cent lindane emulsion.

2 per cent Malathion emulsion

0.5 per cent dieldrin emulsion*

Dead spaces and items (such as fuse boxes) which sprays might damage should be dusted with insecticides:

Silica aerogil

5 per cent chlordane*

3 per cent Malathion

1 per cent dieldrin*

D. Ectoparasites

Ectoparasites cause great misery and may transmit disease. Ectoparasite bites should be disinfected immediately. If the reaction to the bite is severe, a physician should be consulted.

1. Environmental control

Personal hygiene measures to control ectoparasites include frequent bathing, laundering of clothing and laundering bedding.

Dwellings may be protected if the following procedures are carried out:

Vacuum clean floors, rugs and upholstered furniture weekly.

Watch for and eliminate ectoparasites introduced with luggage, clothing and bedding or furniture.

Eliminate cracks and crevices where ectoparasites hide.

Avoid using furniture with wood-to-wood joints and pillows or mattresses with rolled seams.

Keep buildings free of rodents, birds and bats.

Outdoors, keep vegetation cut short along paths and in yards.

2. Chemical control

Lice. Dust infested individuals and contacts with 10 per cent DDT or apply materials prescribed by a physician.

Bedbugs and kissing bugs. Spray cracks and crevices in infested dwellings and furniture with 5 per cent DDT emulsion.

Fleas. Dust infested yards with 5 per cent DDT. Dust infested pets with 3 per cent Malathion. Spray infested houses (floor only) with 1 per cent lindane emulsion.

---

*DO NOT USE CHLORDANE OR DIELDRIN IN BEDROOMS.

Ticks and mites. Spray 2 per cent deodorized Malathion indoors, and dust with 4 per cent Malathion outdoors.

E. Venomous Insects and Arthropods

Persons bitten or stung should be given immediate first aid and, if the reaction is severe, prompt medical care. Venomous insects and arthropods represent a special hazard to the elderly and the infirm.

Clinical manifestations of envenomization include anaphylactic shock, paralysis, necrosis, dermatitis and allergic asthma.

The most dangerous of these insects are the hymenoptera (bees, wasps, etc.), spiders (especially the black widow spider and the brown spider), scorpions, centipedes, millipedes, stinging caterpillars and blister beetles.

1. Environmental control

Educate individuals to avoid venomous creatures. Screen buildings. Keep buildings free of rodents, birds and bats. Keep premises free of litter and debris.

2. Chemical control

Have hymenopteran (bee and wasp) nests treated by professional pest control operators.

Use 1 per cent lindane or 2 per cent chlordane sprays for spiders and webs, hiding places of scorpions, centipedes or millipedes and infestations of stinging caterpillars or blister beetles.

F. Stored Products Pests

The most important of these pests are cockroaches, beetles, moths, ants, mites, silverfish, springtails and psocids.

These pests rob citizens of the United States of more than one billion dollars worth of stored foods annually, contaminating and spoiling far more than they eat. They also damage clothing, rugs and other items; and they cause diseases in man and transmit diseases to man:

> intestinal infestations by fly, beetle and moth larvae
> enteric diseases
> tapeworms
> plague (from fleas in stored grain)
> murine typhus (from fleas in stored grain)
> rickettsialpox (from house mouse mites in stored food)

1. Environment control

Store foods and products in an orderly, sanitary manner in a cool, dry room on racks off the floor. Use old stocks first. Inspect regularly for infested stock, and dispose of any that is found.

2. Chemical control

Spray storerooms with 2.5 per cent DDT suspension (be sure that none gets in or on stored food).

RODENT CONTROL

Rodents are involved in the transmission of more than 25 diseases, among which are

enteric diseases
leptospirosis
plague
trichinosis
rickettsialpox
lymphocytic choriomeningitis

Rodents also destroy food and damage buildings and stored products.

A. Rodent Control Procedures for Nursing Facilities

1. Survey to determine type and degree of infestation.

2. Ectoparasite control to prevent disease transmission by ectoparasites when rodent hosts are killed.

3. Poisoning to reduce rodent populations temporarily.

4. Sanitation to reduce food and harborage.

5. Education to lessen human contact with rodents.

6. Modification to building structure to keep rodents out.

7. *Chemical control:* The usual chemical for rodent ectoparasite control is 10 per cent DDT dust. Rodenticides of choice are

Warfarin
Fumarin
Pival
Pmp
Diphacin.

8. Other considerations: Some residents may come to regard domestic rodents as pets and may object to control operations. Such persons should be handled with consideration, but rodent control should be completed.

9. Safety in insect and rodent control: Insect and rodent control operations present hazards from contact with poisons, machinery and flammable materials. The safest effective pesticide should be used, and control personnel should be constantly aware of the special hazards to nursing facility residents. Only properly trained responsible personnel should be allowed to do insect and rodent control work. Have personnel work in pairs, never alone. Keep bystanders away. Keep chemicals and equipment under constant control so they cannot be stolen or picked up by accident. Require regular maintenance and careful use of equipment.

DISINFECTION AND STERILIZATION

Sterilization is any process that destroys all life—harmful or not, microscopic or not. Few chemicals, if any, as they are used in practical disinfection, are actual sterilization agents.

A *germicide* is any chemical agent that is used to destroy microorganisms. The following are included in this classification:

Bactericide—Any chemical agent that kills bacteria.

Disinfectant—Any chemical agent that is used on inanimate materials and which, although it will not kill bacteria in the spore state, does destroy harmful microorganisms in all other states.

Antiseptic—Any chemical agent that is usually applied to living tissue and which renders microorganisms harmless by either killing them or preventing their growth and reproduction.

Sanitizer — Any chemical agent that is used either to destroy or inactivate contamination which might be objectionable, esthetically or otherwise. Sanitizers are used on materials that have already been cleaned. They leave no harmful residue.

Antimicrobial agent — All kinds of agents that either destroy or inhibit the growth of microorganisms.

DISINFECTANTS

A. Alcohols

Ethyl and propyl alcohols are excellent disinfectants for certain purposes.
1. Properties and characteristics
Evaporate rapidly, leave no residue.

Solvents for some substances (some cleansing capability).

Relatively inexpensive.

Appear to be effective against tubercle bacilli.

Ineffective against spores.

Under certain circumstances, more injurious to human cells than to bacterial cells.

Maximum germicidal effect is obtained only through a narrow range of dilution — concentrations greater than 75 per cent, and those less than 60 per cent, show a marked diminution of germicidal effect.
2. Uses
Preoperative skin preparation.

Sterilization of surgical instruments and thermometers.

B. Chlorine

Chlorine is one of the most useful disinfectants that we have for the disinfection of physically clean surfaces. It is not used in gaseous form, but is available in a variety of organic and inorganic compounds, which are sufficiently unstable to release it in nascent (active) form.
1. Properties and characteristics
Chlorine is most effective in acid solution (pH below 7); somewhat effective in neutral solutions (pH 7); ineffective when used in soap or any other detergent solution which has a high pH.

Chlorine is corrosive (so are many other disinfectants, but proper concentration and handling will mitigate this quality in most applications). It is effective against tubercule bacilli and spores, low-cost and easy to use.
2. Uses
Chlorine-releasing compounds can be used to disinfect many materials, such as floors, mops, bedpans and toilets. Chlorine is a choice disinfectant for use on food-handling equipment.

C. Iodine

Iodine, like chlorine, is a member of the halogen family of elements and has good disinfectant qualities. When iodine is carried by a vehicle known as a surfactant compound, a complex that is known as an iodophor is formed. (The surfactant compound acts as a "go-between" to bring the iodine molecule into close contact with the surface of the material that the surfactant itself touches, and thus promotes chemical action between the iodine and the other material.) Because they are good, iodophors are gaining popularity as disinfectants. They do have a role in the well-balanced sanitation program, but they will not by themselves solve all disinfecting problems.

1. Properties and characteristics

Iodine dissolved in alcohol is an excellent skin antiseptic. Concentrations in the range of 6000 to 20,000 parts of iodine to one million parts of alcohol will destroy the infective capability of spores and of tubercle bacilli.

Iodine carried by a surfactant (forming an iodophor) is most active in the lower pH ranges, and generally must be present in relatively strong concentrations to bring disinfectant activity up to a useful level. Iodophors are nonstaining,* nonirritating,* noncorrosive* and stable.* They are compatible with hard water (up to 1000 p.p.m.) as well as soft water. They are also mildly detergent (have some cleaning ability), but are primarily disinfectant in action, and are less inhibited by the presence of proteinaceous contamination than are either the chlorine-releasing compounds or the quaternary ammonium compounds.

2. Uses

Iodine (alcohol solution)—antiseptic for skin surfaces of patients; disinfectant for heat-sensitive surgical equipment (20,000 p.p.m.).

Iodophors—disinfectant for food service equipment; final disinfectant for fomites.

D. Quaternary Ammonium Compounds

These disinfectants are members of a family of chemically related compounds. A number of agents will inhibit their germicidal activity; and, unfortunately, these inhibiting agents (some of which are soaps, anionic detergents, hexachlorophene and ionic forms of minerals that give water the characteristic of "hardness") are usually included in solutions—accidentally or otherwise—to which it would be convenient to add the ammonium compounds for disinfection purposes. For this reason, the use of these germicides must be tied into overall sanitation practices, because there is every likelihood that haphazard use will vitiate their efficacy.

1. Properties and characteristics

Low toxicity.
Nonirritating.
Good deodorant capability.
Limited virucidal capability.
Ineffective against tubercle bacilli.

2. Uses (on clean surfaces)

Food equipment surfaces.
Food processing plant equipment.
Skin antiseptics.

---

*When used in recommended dilutions in water.

E. Mercurial (And Other Heavy Metal) Compounds

These disinfectant compounds are widely used in hospitals, but there is doubt as to their effectiveness. Because there are germicides of proved utility available, there is no real place for questionable compounds in a modern disinfection program.

F. Formaldehyde (Formalin)

A strong solution of formaldehyde in water is an excellent disinfectant. Formaldehyde and alcohol in water are the most powerful of the commonly available disinfectants.

1. Properties and characteristics
Gives off irritating vapors that limit its use in occupied areas.
Coagulates protein.

2. Uses
Sterilizing instruments.
Disinfecting fomites.

G. Phenols, Bis-Phenols, Halogenated Phenols and Related Compounds

Phenolics are excellent disinfectants. The newer halogenated phenols are particularly powerful, and have the advantage of being nonodorous. The bis-phenols (hexachlorophene, known as G-11; bithional, known also as G5S and as Actamer) are bacteriostats— they must be applied repeatedly and frequently to maintain infection-free conditions. Hexachlorophene, for instance, is of value, not so much as a destroyer of existing organisms but rather because it evaporates slowly and over a period of time inhibits the growth of arriving organisms. Certain members of this bis-phenol group are reported to have the advantage of fewer adverse side effects than the monophenols.

1. Properties and characteristics
Somewhat effective against viruses.
Somewhat effective against tubercle bacilli.
Ineffective against spores.
Caustic (even low concentrations will damage tissues).
Bis-phenols enhance the germicidal properties of formaldehyde and some of the other germicides.
Bis-phenols are slow acting.
The germicidal quality of the bis-phenols is diminished by the presence of organic matter, such as body fluids, pus serum, albumin, milk and similar material. G-11, however, retains sufficient of its germicidal powers, when in the presence of soap, to allow it to have useful practical application.
Hexachlorophene soaps must be used consistently to lower skin flora. Single applications have little effect.

2. Uses
Phenols—disinfecting walls, floors and similar surfaces.
Bis-phenols—skin disinfectants.

H. Pine Oil Compounds

The pleasant odor of these compounds makes them ideal masking agents. Unfortunately, this frequently leads to their being misused for the concealment of unpleasant odors that are emanating from some sort of contamination that should be eliminated by the use of either detergents or germicides or both. Pine oil emulsions do not kill *M. pyogenes var. aureus* (commonly known as Staphylococcus aureus) and therefore cannot be used in place of other disinfectants for general purposes.

1. Properties and characteristics

Capable of killing a variety of microorganisms.
Have detergent qualities.
Nontoxic.
Nonirritating.
Stable.

FACTORS THAT GOVERN THE EFFECTIVENESS OF DISINFECTANTS

The chemical structure of most disinfectants is complex; the mode of action through which they reduce the incidence of infection is not always known. Each type of disinfectant has its own proponents, but even the experts often disagree on which is the best for a particular problem. There are some factors, however, that are fairly common denominators of all disinfectant action. Knowledge of these factors and their effects is an aid in discriminating between valid and fallacious claims.

1. Constituents and their individual properties

Concentration of each ingredient.
Purpose of each ingredient.

2 . Exposure required to inactivate pathogens

Types of pathogens that are inactivated.
Duration of exposure required to inactivate each type.
Temperature range at which a given duration of exposure will inactivate each pathogen.
Concentration of the formulation that will inactivate pathogens under previously prescribed conditions.

3. Other factors

pH of the solvent.   The pH is affected by solutes (such as detergents) that are in solution in the solvent. It is also affected by residues on the surfaces to be disinfected—soluble residues, of course, go into solution when the solvent-disinfectant mixture comes into contact with them.

Organic matter.   Proteinaceous and other materials that are present in the solvent-disinfectant solution, and that are also present as residue on the surfaces to be disinfected, can deleteriously influence the effectiveness of a disinfectant.

Incompatible substances.   These are the chemical substances that are present in the solvent and which can combine chemically with the materials of the formulation to make new compounds that have either fewer or weaker or no disinfectant characteristics. Incompatible substances may include the compounds that cause the characteristic of hardness in water or other impurities, such as residual chlorine or alkali from water treatment.

Properties of materials to be disinfected.   The chemical properties of the materials to be disinfected can determine the advisability of using a formulation that is bacteriologically correct. (Chlorine formulations will attack animal-derived materials.) The physical properties of the materials to be disinfected must be considered—moisture alone will weaken some materials.

4. Side effects

Toxicity.

Irritation.

Discoloration and bleaching.

Allergenic qualities.

Corrosiveness.

Selection Procedures

1. Setting up qualifications

To have utility, any disinfectant must fill certain qualifications, which will depend upon many factors. These qualifications might include the following:

Registration with the U.S. Department of Agriculture.

Ability to control specific pathogens.

Neutrality to materials to be disinfected.

Effectiveness at a given frequency of application.

Compatibility with specific solvents.

Specific admissible degree of toxicity.

2. Screening the disinfectants

Disinfectants should be screened only on the basis of information that is considered reliable, by comparing the qualifications to the properties attributed to each formulation being screened in somewhat the following arrangement:

Identification of product

Brand name.

Name and address of manufacturer (or distributor).

Type of product.

List of ingredients of the formulation by chemical name and percentage (by weight) of each ingredient in the formulation.

Sources of information

U.S.D.A. registered material.

Signed specifications.

Certified results of independent tests.

Instructions for use

Dilutions (for each general application).

Precautions.

Limitations.

Pathogens for which the product is specifically germicidal

Mode of action.

Concentrations required.

Duration of exposure for positive results.

Frequency of application to maintain control.

Method of application.

Pathogens for which the product is noneffective

Toxicity

To forms of life other than pathogens.

In what concentrations.

Cumulative effects.

Corrosiveness

Conditions of temperature and concentration, and conditions in the presence of accelerating and inhibiting agents.

Effect on tissues.

Effect on other materials (equipment, instruments, furniture, etc.).

3. Evaluating the performance of disinfectants

Screened or laboratory and field-proved disinfectants should be evaluated by comparing the results of their performances under actual operating conditions.

Establish control conditions by standardizing all known variables that can affect the performance of each disinfectant. Evaluate the types and densities of the initial bacterial population. Use a candidate disinfectant during a specific period of time, and evaluate the final bacterial population. Re-establish control conditions and allow bacterial population to stabilize at previous levels, then repeat with another candidate disinfectant.

Continual monitoring of disinfectant efficiency is an important part of the selection of disinfectants. Selection must be continuous to cope with changing conditions: The germicidal capacity of the disinfectant may be vitiated by an unrecognized change in procedures, environmental factors or the bacterial population. Continued but ineffective use of the disinfectant can create a false sense of security, and is as dangerous and costly as selecting an ineffective formulation to begin with.

4. The field sanitarian's place in selection follow-up

The field sanitarian should be supported by adequate laboratory services for the evaluation of disinfectants just as he is supported by laboratory capability in water and milk analysis and the evaluation of cleanliness of food handling surfaces.

STERILIZATION

Sterilization is the killing of all forms of microbial life. The most common sterilizing agent is heat; certain gases are also used for this purpose.

Moist Heat Sterilizing

Moist heat is nothing more than heat in the presence of water vapor or, if the temperature is sufficiently high, in the presence of steam. Saturated steam (steam in the presence of water) under pressure — as in an autoclave — is the most dependable means known for the destruction of all forms of microbial life.

Pressure alone (moderate pressure) will not destroy microorganisms. The temperature of saturated steam increases as the pressure of the saturated steam increases. It is the increase in temperature (made possible by the increase in pressure) that destroys microbial life. Because of the situation described in Dalton's Law of Partial Pressures,* the temperature of steam in an autoclave is lower (at the same pressure) if the steam is mixed with air, than if there is only water and steam in the autoclave. For this reason, pressure alone is *not* an indica-

---

*"The total pressure exerted against the interior of a vessel by a given quantity of a mixed gas [in our case, steam and air] enclosed in it, is the sum of the pressures which each of the component gases would exert separately if it were enclosed alone in a vessel of the same volume and at the same temperature."

TABLE 14–2. TEMPERATURE AND PRESSURE ATTAINED IN AN AUTOCLAVE WITH VARYING AMOUNTS OF AIR AND STEAM

AIR AND STEAM	PRESSURE (pounds per sq. inch)	TEMPERATURE (°F.)
No air removed...	15	212
One-third of air removed	15	228
Two-thirds of air removed.............................	15	240
All air removed—saturated steam	15	250

tion of sterilizing capability. All autoclaves should be equipped with thermometers, and these, rather than pressure gauges, should be relied upon in measuring time-temperature combinations for sterilization purposes. *If air happens to get trapped in a steam sterilizer, it is possible to have "correct" sterilizing pressures without actually attaining sterilizing temperatures* (Table 14–2.)

Twelve minutes is the shortest time in which effective sterilization will take place at a temperature of 250° F. Fifteen pounds per square inch of pressure (gauge) is necessary for saturated steam to reach a temperature of 250° F. This temperature must be maintained *in all parts* of the material being sterilized for the full 12 minutes. If the temperature in an autoclave is increased, the time during which material to be sterilized must be subjected to the temperature may be reduced (Table 14–3).

Dry Heat Sterilizing

Many materials cannot be sterilized by steam because of their physical properties. Such materials may, however, often be sterilized by dry heat without affecting them adversely.

Hot air ovens use dry heat to sterilize. To be effective, they must have certain design characteristics: They should use about 520 watts of electricity per cubic foot of sterilizing temperature (320° F.) in not more than 30 minutes of operation. At no point in the sterilizing space should the temperature vary more than 2° F. from the operating temperature of the oven.

Temperature-time relationships in dry heat sterilizing are the same as in moist-heat sterilizing (Table 14–4).

TABLE 14–3. TIME-TEMPERATURE RELATIONSHIPS FOR MOIST HEAT STERILIZATION

TIME (minutes)	TEMPERATURE (°F.)
2	270
8	257
12	250
18	245

TABLE 14–4. TIME-TEMPERATURE RELATIONSHIPS FOR
DRY HEAT STERILIZATION

TIME (hours)	TEMPERATURE (° F.)
1...	340
2...	320
2½...	300
3...	285
6...	250

Gas Sterilizing

Ethylene dioxide is now used as a sterilizing agent. In liquid form, the compound is flammable, but will not detonate. The vapor state of the compound, of course, burns and also combines explosively with air. Because of this quality, it is mixed with an inert gas such as carbon dioxide for marketing.

CHAPTER FIFTEEN

HOUSEKEEPING SERVICES

Housekeeping and maintenance service must be provided to maintain a sanitary and comfortable environment.

Cleanliness is a requisite to the healthfulness of any environment. The importance of the biological aspect of cleanliness is equal to, if not greater than, the mere physical and esthetic considerations of cleanliness. Housekeeping is the business of keeping premises, equipment and facilities clean and orderly.

In the absence of a trained housekeeper, the housekeeping is performed by aides, orderlies or, in many cases, handyman janitors. Sufficient personnel must be provided to maintain the interior and exterior of the facility in a safe, clean, orderly and attractive manner. Supervisory personnel must have a complete knowledge of the theory, practice, methods and tools of housekeeping. They must be able to impart their knowledge to others, instruct in supporting skills and recognize problems and solve them.

Personnel providing direct nursing care must not be assigned housekeeping duties.

BASIC CONSIDERATIONS IN THE HOUSEKEEPING PROGRAM

Built-in sanitation is important in keeping a building clean. Factors of importance in design of the facility are the availability of utility rooms, dirty linen storage, hopper sinks and bedpan rinsers and flushers.

Housekeeping personnel, using the accepted practices and procedures, must keep the facility free from offensive odors, from accumulations of dirt, rubbish and dust and from safety hazards. Floors must be cleaned regularly, and polishes must provide a non-slip finish. Throw or scatter rugs must not be used except for non-slip entrance mats.

Walls and ceilings must be maintained free of cracks and falling plaster and must be cleaned and painted regularly.

Deodorizers must not be used to cover up odors caused by unsanitary conditions or poor housekeeping practices.

Storage areas, attics and cellars must be kept safe and free from the accumulation of extraneous materials such as refuse, discarded furniture and old newspapers. Combustibles such as cleaning rags and compounds must be kept in closed metal containers.

Grounds must be kept free from refuse and litter.

NUMBER AND TYPE OF PATIENTS

Patients' conditions will vary from healthy to chronically ill, from fully mobile to completely immobile, from self-sufficient to fully dependent. A large number of patients will be in the higher age brackets. They will be ill and consequently susceptible to infection of all sorts. Some patients will be incontinent of feces or urine or both.

MEDICAL CARE OFFERED

A wide variety of situations that affect housekeeping practice will occur. There will be patients with draining lesions, patients requiring indwelling catheters, patients who have colostomies and patients confined to bed who have decubitus ulcers (bed sores); and some patients might have staphylococcus infections. All these patients present special problems in sanitation and disinfection.

SIZE AND QUALITY OF STAFF

The responsibility for supervising housekeeping falls upon the administrator, and it is his responsibility to select, train and supervise all of the unskilled personnel who perform the housekeeping duties.

The system and method in housekeeping of division of labor increases efficiency and economy. Under proper supervision, unskilled personnel can perform discrete parts of more complex tasks. The division of labor enables the standardizing of simplified tasks.

A work schedule should be developed for each employee. The tasks should be arranged in consecutive order from the beginning of a work period to its end. That period may be a day, a week, a month or an even longer period of time. The purposes of this schedule are as follows:

To give the employee a reliable list of the duties he is expected to perform.

To insure that time is provided for each employee's duties.

To fix responsibility for all the tasks that are performed.

To enable the administrator to better oversee the operation.

To provide a basis for an estimate and review of the work load.

To prevent excessive lost motion for new employees.

The administrator should develop, by the following procedures, work schedules containing information for housekeeping employees:

Survey the cleaning and maintenance needs. Check all areas, omiting or neglecting no activity.

Indicate the frequency of cleaning each piece of equipment and every type of surface.

Set time limits for the execution of each task by experience, observation and testing.

Indicate the best time during the work day for each task, and include time for meals, rest periods and recreation periods. Indicate duties each employee should be responsible for as well as the locations in which these duties will be carried out.

Consolidate all duties assigned to each individual on a separate form; this is the individual's work schedule. Note on the work schedule other responsibilities assigned to the employee, such as emergency activities and special assistance to other employees.

Jobs

A *description* of each employee's job should be formulated. It should include
The job name.
Names of tasks, such as sweeping, window washing, polishing brass.
Degree of capability required for each task, including physical requirements and mental and educational requirements.
Degree of proficiency.
The level of judgment and initiative required.
Special qualifications, if any.

Training.   The training program must meet the needs of both the workers and the administrator. A clean, healthful environment is necessary to a good operation, which is in turn dependent upon efficient training. Areas that training improves are,

Among workers:
Efficiency
Productivity
Morale
Initiative
Interest
Among administrators:
Supervision
Surveillance
Cleaning procedures
Inspection
Evaluation of products

There are direct economic advantages to training in the reduction of operating costs and the reduction in labor turnover.

Tasks

A cleaning task is a single kind of operation in a particular area, such as sweeping a specific hallway or washing windows on a particular floor.

Give each task a name that specifically applies to it and to no other task. List the tasks.

Certain facts must be determined about each of the listed tasks:

The reason for performing it.

Methods used to perform it, the actions necessary and their sequence.

The efficiency of the existing method. List possibilities for improvement, and eliminate all but the best method obtained by evaluation.

The materials and equipment needed in the execution of the task.

Estimate of the time required to perform the task.

The priority rating of the task—necessity of the task as compared with other tasks.

Describe the task in simple terms, utilizing the same nomenclature and sequence in all task descriptions.

Measuring Results

Measuring the results of cleaning operation is difficult. The best method of evaluating this is not one of measuring cleanliness but of measuring the opposite, the degree of contamination. Uniform standards for measurements must be established. Standards must be set for appearance, odor and bacterial contamination, including the kind of bacteria and the quantity of each type of bacteria. The finish of each surface, permeability of the surface, texture of the surface, condition of the surface, results of wear and results of exposure and orderliness should also be measured.

Methods

The *empirical* method of measuring cleanliness is by use of rating forms and check lists.

The most reliable *physical* method of measuring cleanliness is the proper use of paper swab and light meter technique. Standard paper swab is rubbed on a surface to be graded. The soiled swab is then compared to an unused swab. By use of a light meter it measures the difference in the light that is reflected by the two swabs.

The *biological* methods of measuring cleanliness on surfaces are swabbing, rinsing and contact (spot plate—plate can be incubated directly). For air, the following products are used to evaluate contamination by sweeping, dusting, vacuuming and the like: Anderson sampler, slit sampler, membrane filters, sieve sampler and settling plate.

Results of measurements

Unless results are reproducible they are of no practical value. Used correctly, grading forms and check lists can be most useful for the measurement of housekeeping efficiency and quality. Other tools, as previously stated, are the paper swab and light meter.

PEST CONTROL

The facility must be maintained free from insects and rodents. A pest control program must be in operation in the facility. Pest control services may be provided by the maintenance personnel of the facility or by contract with a pest control company.

The least toxic and least flammable effective insecticides and rodenticides should be used. They should be stored in non-patient areas and in non-food preparation and storage areas. Poisons must be under lock. Windows and doors must be screened during insect breeding seasons.

Garbage and trash must be stored in an area separate from those used for the preparation and storage of food and must be removed from the premises in conformity with state and local practices. Containers must be cleaned regularly.

Further details may be found in Chapter 14, "Physical Environment."

LINEN SUPPLY

The facility must have available at all times the quantity of linens essential for the proper care and comfort of patients. Linens must be handled, stored and processed so as to control the spread of infection. Linen supply must be at least three times the usual occupancy.

Clean linens and clothing must be stored in clear, dry, dust-free areas easily accessible to the nurses' station. Soiled linens must be stored in separate well ventilated areas and must not be permitted to accumulate in the facility. Soiled linens and clothing must be stored separately in suitable bags or containers. It must not be sorted, laundered, rinsed or stored in bathrooms, patient rooms, kitchens or food storage areas.

Further details may be found under Chapter 16, "Laundry Services."

TABLE 15–1. HOUSEKEEPING EQUIPMENT

MANUAL EQUIPMENT	
1. Buckets and Wringers	Mop bucket, dolly and wringer should be cleaned daily . . . Clean and oil casters on dolly and replace casters when defective . . . Oil all working parts of wringer regularly . . . Replace bumper strips on dolly when necessary.
2. Wet Mops	Do not twist mop when wringing . . . Clean mop, rinse and wring out after each use . . . Use mop holders when storing mops so mop heads do not touch floor . . . Use proper size mop wringer.
3. Window Squeegees	Wash and wipe dry after each use . . . Adjust blade tension or replace blades as required . . . A squeegee is a professional tool . . . treat it as such.
4. Sponges and Chamois	Wash and rise out after each use . . . Store on rack to allow for complete drying.
5. Dust Mops	Spray dust treatment with electric sprayer . . . Place in covered container . . . Do not use on wet or oily floors . . . Replace mop head when soiled . . . Launder soiled mop heads, dry and re-treat.

TABLE 15–1.   HOUSEKEEPING EQUIPMENT—Continued

FLOOR MACHINES

1. Mount brushes by hand	Make sure that switch is off... Do not run machine over brush and attach starting motor... Start machine only when brush is securely locked on... Use proper brush for the job.
2. Care for electric cord	Prevent machine from running over electric cord... Inspect cord frequently for damage, fraying, etc.... Wipe cord after each use with damp cloth and dry thoroughly... Wind cord loosely around hooks on machine when not in use... Remove plug from outlet carefully—do not jerk cord.
3. Schedule periodic inspection	Should be done by qualified electricians or maintenance men... Don't allow minor repairs to grow into major overhauls... Scheduled inspections will prevent "down time" and costly repair bills.
4. Care for brushes	Remove brushes from machine when not in use... Hang brushes up or lay on shelf with bristles up... Wash brushes when soiled in warm detergent solution... Do not saturate wood backs... Dry with bristles up... Keep adapter plates tightened.
5. Clean and lubricate	Wipe machine with cloth dipped in germicidal-detergent solution... Keep motor and electrical equipment dry... Oil mechanical moving parts and lubricate motor... Polish all metal parts... Store in safe location.

WET PICK-UP VACUUM CLEANERS

1. Use correctly	Start vacuuming next to machine... Work away from machine, so that hose and cord follow you... Do not back into machine... Use proper tools.
2. Care for electric cord	Wipe cord with damp cloth after each use and dry thoroughly... Inspect cord regularly for damage, fraying, etc.... Prevent machine from running over cord... Wind cord loosely around top of machine when not in use.
3. Schedule periodic inspection	Secure needed adjustments or repairs... Have work done by qualified electricians or maintenance men... Neglect of minor repairs or adjustments will cause major "down time" and expense.
4. Clean and lubricate	Wipe machine inside and out with cloth dipped in germicidal-detergent solution... Empty and dry tank after each use... Clean and oil casters... Lubricate motor according to manufacturer's directions... Store vacuum with top removed for thorough drying.

CHAPTER SIXTEEN

LAUNDRY SERVICES

The laundry receives contaminated washable goods from virtually every operation in the facility. Proper procedures can facilitate the elimination of cross-infection throughout the operation. The laundering operation is an important factor in controlling contamination in the environment, and it is the bulwark in the program aimed at preventing the spread of infection.

Proper laundry operation prevents the spread of contamination and contributes to its elimination. The proper processing of laundered materials can prevent the fabrics from becoming irritating to the skin.

For employees, the proper handling of contaminated linen can prevent exposure to infective agents. Adequately controlled working conditions can do likewise.

HANDLING OF DIRTY LAUNDRY

Blankets, pillows and other such items should never be transferred from one patient to another without having first been cleaned and sanitized. All washable items should be handled and stored as follows:

Unnecessary agitation of patients' soiled clothing and of linens during bed changes must be avoided because it increases the possibility of spreading airborne infective agents.

Each patient's soiled clothing should be kept in an individual clothes container until it is delivered to a dirty storage area or to the laundering area.

Soiled linens must always be transported to the dirty storage or laundry area in closed hampers or bags. Separate identifiable bags for isolation laundry must be used. If laundry chutes are used the soiled linens must be enclosed in suitable bags.

216

There should be no contact between clean and soiled linen and clothing at any point, either in transport or in storage areas.

Carts and bags used to transport clean items should never be used for soiled linen and clothing.

A separate room should be reserved for the sorting and storage of soiled linen and clothing.

Extra blankets distributed during cold weather should never be returned for redistribution without first having been cleaned and sanitized.

HANDLING OF CLEAN LAUNDRY

Clean articles should be bundled and wrapped. The bundles should be moved from the laundry in carts, bags or other containers. These laundry containers should be cleaned frequenly—if they have washable inserts or removable plasticized basket liners, these should be removed and cleaned at frequent intervals.

Clean goods should be stored properly as soon as they have been processed and packaged in the laundry.

Storage areas (linen closets, etc.) for clean goods should never be used for any other purpose; they should not become catchalls for personal belongings, cleaning compounds, bed guard rails or similar items.

When clean linen is removed from storage for distribution, only the articles that are needed in an area should be carried into that area. For example, only the bed linen that is actually needed in a patient's room should go into that room.

PHYSICAL ASPECTS OF THE LAUNDRY FACILITY

The laundry must be laid out and its equipment arranged so that the process will not only maintain the proper separation of soiled and clean items, but also will prevent the mingling—or contamination by airflow or other factors—of items in any of the various stages of processing.

DIRTY LAUNDRY ASSEMBLY AND SORTING ROOM

The soiled linen assembly and sorting room is the "dirtiest" part of the laundry. This room should be adjacent to the washing area so soiled goods that are not in containers or bags will not have to pass through other areas of the laundry (or of the nursing facility) as they are taken to the washers; and it must be separate, and both structurally and mechanically closed off, to keep lint, dust and bacteria from being spread throughout other areas of the laundry and the nursing facility.

WASHING AND EXTRACTING AREA

The physical facilities and their arrangement should permit soiled articles to be loaded into washers with a minimum of handling and agitation to avoid contaminating the air and, through the air, other equipment and articles in the laundry. This is particularly important because air is drawn through the extractors while they are operating and, if this air is contaminated, the washed items will be recontaminated. Washers and extractors are in the laundering area proper, but they should not be in the same area in which tumbling, ironing and folding take place.

Under no condition should soiled articles come into contact with either finished or partly finished articles.

FINISHING AREA

This area (where the laundry is dried, tumbled, ironed or pressed and folded) is sometimes referred to as the "heat barrier." It should be between the washing-extractor area and the clean articles storage room. The heat used in the finishing operations helps to sanitize the washed laundry. This heat is the last sanitizing agent that is applied. After this process, the clean laundry should be rigorously safeguarded against recontamination.

CLEAN STORAGE

The storage area for the clean laundry should be apart from the soiled laundry and sorting area and from the washing area. It should be a closed room that affords maximum protection against contamination. No sewage lines should run overhead through this room, because they could be a source of contamination if a leak were to develop. This area should be well ventilated to prevent condensation of moisture on the walls, shelves and stored articles.

The storage shelves should be located well above the floor so that stored laundry will not be contaminated by cleaning operations such as mopping floors.

VENTILATION

The movement of air in and out of the laundering area is important because the effect of precautions taken in the various stages of processing can be negated if laundry becomes contaminated with airborne bacteria at any stage of processing, particularly after it goes through finishing procedures. Some nursing homes cope with the problem of airborne contaminants by conducting the laundering operation in a building that is separate and far removed from the nursing home proper. Those facilities which do not approach the problem in this way should comply with the following requirements:

In the laundering area, the direction of airflow should be directly opposite to the direction of the flow of the articles being processed. The air from the finishing and clean storage area should pass into the washing area and then out of the structure.

The dirty laundry storage and sorting room should be vented directly to the outside, and air should be removed from it at a faster rate than air is being removed from the surrounding laundering area. The partial vacuum thus created in the sorting and dirty storage room prevents the air in this room from going into other parts of the laundering area.

Laundry chutes should not open directly into the laundering area because they would be, in effect, direct air passages from a contaminated area to other parts of the nursing home.

LAUNDERING PROCEDURES

This outline on laundering procedures only highlights the important aspects of sanitation. For detailed information on laundering practice, the American Hospital Association's manual of Operation of Hospital Laundry is recommended.

PERSONAL AND ENVIRONMENTAL HYGIENE

Hand Washing

Hand washing facilities (soap and hot water) should be available in the laundry area. Use of hexachlorophene soap is urged as one means of protecting laundry workers against work-acquired infections as well as preventing them from infecting others.

Toilet Facilities

There should be toilet facilities located in the laundry area.

Uniforms

Laundry workers should not wear street clothing when they are working; uniforms should be provided for them. Workers who handle soiled goods must change their uniforms and wash their hands each time before they handle clean laundry. Other workers handling only clean goods should have a clean uniform daily.

Uniforms should not be worn outside the laundry area.

HOUSEKEEPING

Housekeeping within the laundering area is of prime importance.

Floors, walls, ceilings, pipes and equipment must be kept clean and free of lint and grease. Wet vacuum cleaning and other cleaning procedures must be carried out on a regular schedule. Floors should be wet-mopped and sanitized daily. Cleaning must be done in a way that minimizes the possibility of contaminating laundry.

The responsibility for housekeeping in the laundering area should be given to a specific person so it will not be neglected through oversight or misunderstanding. This activity should be shown on that person's work schedule, and the jobs that it includes should appear in the procedure manual of the nursing home. In the larger facilities, this activity is one of the responsibilities of the housekeeping department.

SORTING DIRTY LAUNDRY

Soiled linens should be handled as little as possible; sorting should be simple and brief. Laundry workers should be instructed in practices that will both safeguard their health and prevent the spread of infective agents to the other parts of the nursing home.

WASHING

The washing process should effectively sanitize the laundry. Proper washing procedures call for water at a temperature of 165° F. or above, and an exposure of soiled articles to the water at this temperature for 25 or more minutes. This treatment effectively disinfects the laundry. If low temperatures must be used in laundering processes, a sufficient quantity of a suitable chemical disinfectant should be added to the wash water to insure that the process is effectively bactericidal.

WASHING FORMULAS

Factors that must be considered in establishing washing formulas are as follows:

Type and color of goods being washed, which controls the choice of detergents or soaps, the use of bleaches, the temperature of the water and the use of chemical disinfectants.

Kind and amount of soil, which controls the amount of suds, the use of water softeners (to some extent), the choice of detergents or soaps, the temperature of the water and the number of rinses.

Hardness of the water and the equipment available, which controls the amount of suds, the use of water softeners, the choice of detergents or soaps, the number of rinses and the degree of souring.

The following is a partial list of laundry agents acceptable when used in the manner and concentration recommended by the manufacturer:

Sours

Sodium acid fluoride	Fluosilicic acid
Ammonium acid fluoride	Oxalic acid
Zinc silico fluoride	Acetic acid
Sodium silico fluoride	Formic acid
Ammonium silico fluoride	

Bleaches	*Germicides*
Sodium hypochlorite	Sodium hypochlorite — bleach
Calcium hypochlorite	Calcium hypochlorite — bleach
Sodium perborate	Phenolic compounds — disinfectant
Hydrogen peroxide	Chloramine-T — bleach
Chloramine-T	Quaternary ammonium compounds (hard water–compatible)

The above agents, when used in concentrations applicable to commercial laundry work, are beneficial in the disinfection of laundry items.

TABLE 16–1. TYPICAL LAUNDERING FORMULAS
(Time and Temperature)
LIGHT SOIL WASHING FORMULA

OPERATION	TEMPERATURE (° F.)	TIME (minutes)
1. Suds	120	5
2. Suds and bleach	140–160	5
3. Rinse	160	3
4. Rinse	160	3
5. Rinse	140	3
6. Blue	100	4
7. Sour	100	4

MODERATE SOIL WASHING FORMULA

OPERATION	TEMPERATURE (° F.)	TIME (minutes)
1. Suds	120	5
2. Suds	140–160	5
3. Suds and bleach	160	5
4. Rinse	160	3
5. Rinse	160–180	3
6. Rinse	160	3
7. Rinse	140	3
8. Blue	100	4
9. Sour	100	4

HEAVY SOIL WASHING FORMULA

OPERATION	TEMPERATURE (° F.)	TIME (minutes)
1. Suds	120	5
2. Suds	140–160	5
3. Suds and alkali	160	5
4. Suds and bleach	160	5
5. Rinse	160	3
6. Rinse	160–180	3
7. Rinse	160–180	3
8. Rinse	140	3
9. Blue	100	4
10. Sour	100	4

WOOL BLANKET WASHING FORMULA

OPERATION	TEMPERATURE (° F.)	TIME (minutes)
1. Suds	90–100	5
2. Suds	90–100	5
3. Rinse	90–100	3
4. Rinse	90–100	3
5. Rinse	90–100	3
6. Sour	90–100	5
7. Germicide	90–100	7

FINISHING CLEAN LAUNDRY

Finishing operations should be carried on in a clean and sanitary environment to avoid all possibility of recontaminating the washed articles. The finished laundry should be free of dirt, irritating chemicals and pathogenic organisms.

With the exception of woolen materials, all laundry should be finished by ironing or tumbling or both.

Flatwork should be ironed at a temperature of 328° F. All other ironing and pressing should be carried out at a temperature of 320° F. or higher.

Laundry should be tumbled (fluff-dried) at the maximum temperature permitted by the goods. Tumblers which draw air through coils that are heated to 328° F. have an inside temperature of 250° F. or more. (This is the same temperature that is obtained in an autoclave operating at 15 p.s.i.).

TRANSPORTING

Washable goods, depending on their condition or stage of processing, should be transported in one of three different sets of vehicles.

There must be separate carts, hampers or such used solely for soiled goods.

Vehicles that are used to convey goods from the washer to the extractor, and from the extractor to the tumbler (or other equipment in the finishing area), should not go beyond the finishing areas.

Clean laundry should be transported to its storage area and to its point of use in conveyances that are used exclusively for clean articles.

All articles that are being transported from clean storage to their points of use should be covered to protect them from contamination.

CLEANING MATTRESSES AND PILLOWS

When a weight is placed on either a mattress or a pillow, the resulting compression of the stuffing forces air out through the ticking. When the weight is removed, the expansion of the stuffing sucks air in though the ticking. Microorganisms are sucked in and pushed out with the air; airborne infective agents can be spread in this way. If swabs from an unprotected mattress are cultured, large numbers of microorganisms, including those typical of the resident who last used the mattress, are usually found.

Mattresses

The care of mattresses is a problem because they cannot be washed and disinfected. However, both mattresses and patients can be protected from airborne contaminants by putting mattresses in either plastic or other composition covers. These covers must be cleaned periodically when the same patient uses them over a long period of time and whenever necessary if they are used by an incontinent patient. They should always be cleaned before being transferred from one mattress to another or from one patient to another.

The procedure for cleaning a mattress that has been enclosed in a plastic or other composition cover is as follows:

TABLE 16–2. DAILY LINEN REQUIREMENTS PER PATIENT

ITEM	EACH RESIDENT DAILY	ADDITIONAL FOR INCONTINENT CASES	TOTAL
Bottom sheet	1	2	3
Top sheet	1	1	2
Draw sheet	1	3	4
Bedspread	1	0	1
Towel	2	0	2
Washcloth	1	0	1

Remove the cover from the mattress and wash both sides of the cover in a detergent solution.

Rinse the cover thoroughly with clear water.

Sanitize the cover with an iodophor or other suitable germicide.

Wipe the cover dry (on both sides) with a clean cloth, and hang the cover in a well ventilated place.

Use a brush that has been dampened in an alkaline cleaner and quaternary ammonium compound solution to clean the mattress. Give special attention to seams, corners and edges. Clean both sides of the mattress.

Let the mattress and its cover dry completely before putting the cover back on the mattress.

Pillows

Pillows can be washed and disinfected with special equipment; they can be sent to a commercial laundry for cleaning and disinfection; or, if proper equipment is available, they can be cleaned in the facility. Pillows that have been protected by plastic or other composition covers can be cleaned in the same way as mattresses that are similarly protected.

CLEAN LAUNDRY STORAGE CAPACITIES

Regardless of the type of laundering service that is adopted, the facility must have space and equipment for handling clean and soiled goods.

TABLE 16–3. LINEN REQUIREMENTS PER BED

ITEM	MINIMUM NUMBER IN GOOD CONDITION
Sheets	8
Pillow cases	6
Bed blankets	2½
Bedspreads	1½
Washcloths	4
Hand towels	4
Bath towels	5
Bath blankets	1½

CHAPTER SEVENTEEN

DISASTER PLAN

It is of paramount importance that a fully organized and implemented disaster plan be written and practiced regularly by all personnel. The administrative authority should be the individual responsible for signaling the operation of the disaster plan, including announcing the emergency and its nature to all key personnel.

The following personnel should be immediately called:

Administrator
Director of nurses
Engineer
Administrative physician

PROCEDURES

The charge nurses in all units should be responsible for arranging to have all ambulatory patients brought to a central holding station and for making them comfortable pending further relocation.

Non-ambulatory patients should be prepared for evacuation from their rooms in the event of necessity.

A complete census of patients should immediately be made to determine their location and identity.

Should the emergency be in the form of an attack by a foreign adversary, ambulatory patients should immediately be taken to the prescribed shelter area and bed patients should be moved into a central sheltered area.

Light-security in the evening should be put into effect, securing all windows and doorways from outside light.

Should the emergency occur during evening and bedtime hours, bed clothing should be made available to patients so that they may sleep during the emergency.

The administrative physician should make every effort to contact as many attending physicians as possible and alert them to the possibility of need for their services.

Direct contact should be made with the weather service, and the emergency radio system should be prepared for use in the event it goes on the air.

Following the emergency, the same persons (such as the charge nurse) responsible for the initial relocation of patients should also be responsible for their relocation in normal housing areas.

The administration, director of nurses and administrative physician should perform a survey of all patient areas to determine the condition of patients and condition of nursing units.

The administrative person in charge of the entire operation should be responsible for completing a total and complete report of the emergency, particularly noting any procedural errors to be corrected.

WATER SUPPLY EMERGENCY

Should a water shortage come about, the administrative authority should establish the priority of usage — internal use in the care of patients and drinking, cooking and emergency use.

The water supply authority should immediately be notified.

The engineer should proceed immediately to close those valves unnecessary in the priority use of water and should assure the availability of water in essential areas such as boilers.

Water should not be used by any personnel who may not need it immediately to protect health and are in a position to seek water outside of the facility.

The fire department should be notified immediately and requested to determine whether water is sufficiently available in the event of fire.

Washing and bathing should be discontinued temporarily.

Should it appear that the water shortage will continue beyond several hours, immediate steps should be taken to have water supplied to the facility by mobile carrier.

HEATING EMERGENCY

During the months of the year when the outside temperature falls below 60° F., it is important to have a program for the comfort of patients and protection of the plant and its equipment in the event of a breakdown in the heating system. The procedures in this program should be as follows:

The key personnel in the disaster plan should be immediately called.

The administrative authority on duty should be in charge.

The heating contractor should be immediately requested to inspect the system to determine the possible duration of the heat loss. Should it be expected to last more than six hours, arrangements should be made to evacuate as many patients either to another building or to another location which does not have the heating problem.

Patients remaining in the facility should be issued additional blankets and other protection to assure their comfort and prevent exposure.

The engineer should make immediate arrangements to protect the plant and equipment, including plumbing, water lines, drains and other solution-carrying equipment, to assure prevention of freezing.

Fire extinguishers should be made ready for immediate use in the event of need for them.

Arrangements should be made immediately with the heating contractor to either repair or replace the defective parts of the heating system.

Should the heating system be tied in with the cooking system and other services to patients, arrangements should be immediately made available to assure the continuity of the total care of the patients.

The administrative physician should contact as many attending physicians as possible in order to assure continued care and treatment to patients, particularly during the time of emergency.

CHAPTER EIGHTEEN

ACCIDENT PREVENTION

Accidents do not just happen: they are caused. They are rarely the result of a single factor, but rather a combination of factors operating in a certain sequence to produce sudden, unintentional events which cause injury or property damage.

In the nursing facility, the additional human factors of age, chronic illness and disability increase the accident potential. This emphasizes the need for maximum awareness of safety on the part of the administration and employees and as much awareness as can be imparted to the patients.

A well planned and well executed safety program is essential to the operation. In order to accomplish this, a sincere interest and around-the-clock surveillance by the administrator and supervisory personnel are essential.

Accident problems, the causative factors and types of accidents must be thoroughly understood by the staff for an effective program to exist. This understanding can be accomplished by training sessions in safety.

CAUSATIVE FACTORS IN ACCIDENTS

Causative factors leading to accidents are classified as environmental and human. Control of environmental factors, such as property, equipment and safe surroundings, will not in itself prevent accidents. The human factors — sensory, motor, emotional, attitudinal and those factors related to lack of knowledge or experience — are common to all classes and types of accidents.

ENVIRONMENTAL FACTORS

Environmental factors have to do with the design of the physical plant, its maintenance and its operation. Accidents can sometimes be attributed to the presence of specific hazards. Therefore, the number of these hazards should be kept as low as possible to assure a safe, adequately designed physical plant and one that is properly maintained and operated. The extended care facility administrator should consult with health officials, the fire department, the building inspector, the plumbing inspector, a qualified architect or building designer and state or local officials who might assist him.

Studies have proven that over 65 per cent of all patient accidents in extended care facilities occur in bedrooms. Over 13 per cent occur in the bathrooms. Over 11 per cent occur in hallways. Over 6 per cent occur in the day or activity rooms, and the remaining 5 per cent occur in other areas of the facility.

Injuries resulting from these accidents are attributable in over 40 per cent of the cases to slipping or tripping on floors; 25 per cent of accidents are the result of falls from beds.

HUMAN FACTORS

Despite maintenance of the safest environments possible, accidents occur because of the human element.

Accidents involving *physical* factors may be caused by

Visual abnormalities, such as night blindness, uncorrected visual defects or impairments of vision.

Inability to recognize sounds or odors suggesting the existence of dangerous situations.

Instability of the extremities due to age, disability, illness, medication or other factors.

Acute physical conditions, such as fainting, convulsion, heart attack or cerebral hemorrhage, or other illness.

Physical weakness due to age and impairment of motor functions.

Mental factors leading to accidents may include

Emotional reactions such as fear, anger, frustration, grief, worry.

Poor judgment.

Ignorance in recognizing hazards.

Refusal to accept assistance.

Inability to focus attention.

Forgetfulness.

Staff attitude.   Indifference or neglect by the staff is conducive to higher accident rates. Staff members must be constantly alert and must act responsibly to prevent patients from entering hazardous areas or performing unsafe acts.

PROMOTING A HAZARD-FREE ENVIRONMENT

Handrails on both sides of halls or walkways and on steps both inside and outside of facility are necessary.

Use of ramps should be encouraged. Stairs should be kept clean and free of litter. They should have easily accessible light switches at the top and bottom.

There should be sufficient light on steps to eliminate glare and shadows. Both top and bottom of steps should be lighted.

Flush thresholds at doorways are essential.

Use of scatter rugs should be prohibited.

Rugs or carpets must be securely fastened in patient rooms.

No slippery wax or moisture should be present on floors.

Variable-height beds that allow for sitting height as well as beds that are not easily moved are necessary.

Footstools, cords, low furniture and other obstacles must be removed from the middle of the floor.

Well balanced chairs in good repair and of proper height for individual patients must be used.

Sufficient light for all sections of the room is necessary. Light fixtures must be properly grounded and switches must be close to the bed.

No appliances with open flame or unguarded hot surfaces may be permitted.

Properly ventilated heating units are essential.

All electrical equipment must be Underwriters' Laboratories-approved. Gas units must be approved by the American Gas Association and installed according to local codes.

Flammable liquids such as alcohol, pressurized sprays and fuel oils must be removed.

PATIENTS' BATHROOMS

Bathroom floors must have nonskid surfaces. Rubber suction mats or safety grip strips should be provided for tubs and showers.

Floors must be dry. Mop all water or other spilled liquids from floors promptly.

Grab-bars and handrails for commodes, tubs, showers and walls must be properly anchored.

Only properly grounded electrical equipment may be used, away from the tub and shower area.

Room heaters must be properly installed. There should be no temporary heaters.

Thermostatically controlled water should be at 110° F., maximum.

There should be no medicine cabinets.

PATIENT BEHAVIOR

All staff members should be aware of the need for older persons to
Take care in walking and avoid long strides.
Avoid the use of high-heeled shoes; but wear shoes, not slippers.
Refrain from lifting or moving heavy objects.
Refrain from reaching beyond normal height. This may cause loss of balance.
Refrain from attempting to stand when feeling dizzy or faint.
Use extra caution on stairs, especially if wearing bifocal glasses.
Refrain from taking a hot bath or getting in or out of tub alone.
Leave bathroom or bedroom doors unlocked.
Call for assistance when needed.
Refrain from climbing on unsteady objects.
Refrain from smoking in bed unless supervised.

TYPES OF ACCIDENTS

Falls

Over 50 per cent of all patient accidents are falls. This is more than three times as many as from any other single cause.

Burns

Burns due to fire, hot surfaces and hot liquids, and other injuries associated with fire, are the second greatest cause of death in accidents.

Poisoning

Prevention of this type of accident is based on proper use and control of poisonous materials and is the direct responsibility of the extended care facility staff. This includes protection of drugs, housekeeping supplies and insecticides. Proper installation and operation of gas burning equipment is also necessary to prevent injuries by gas poisoning or asphyxiation.

Electric Shocks

Overloading of electrical systems, connections of unapproved or defective appliances and similar abuses of the use of electrical energy cause fires which result in injury and loss of life. Mild electric shocks may cause persons to jump or otherwise lose their balance, causing injury to themselves or others.

Injuries from Cutting and Piercing

Razors, pocket knives and scissors are the items with which patients are most likely to come into contact. Care and precaution should be exercised in the issuing of these articles to patients.

Others

Patients being struck by other patients, for example, by hand, walking cane or crutches, can cause injuries such as fractures, lacerations and severe bruises. A partial solution might be the classifying of patients as to likes and dislikes in rooming habits, associates, eating habits and recreational interests. Safety education and supervised walks tend to reduce these abuses.

CHAPTER NINETEEN

FIRE SAFETY

In order to prevent the development of conditions predisposing to fire, and in order to minimize death and injury if one does develop, there must be an understanding of the four components of fire safety: the building; the contents of the building; the people in the building; and the provision for fire detection and control.

EXITS

One of the most important factors in preventing death and injury is the ability to safely and rapidly evacuate all patients and staff from the building. Emergency situations may occur other than fire which call for also prompt evacuation of the building. Major considerations are the following:

Exits must be unlocked and must open outwardly.

All floors should have at least two exits per floor, remote from each other and reasonably equidistant from the center.

There should be an exit from every patient location, and there should be one not further than 50 feet from the farthest patient area.

Exits must be properly lighted with exit signs.

Exits in halls must be free from obstruction.

Orderliness is dependent, of course, upon a tested evacuation plan known to all members of the extended care facility.

FIRE AND SMOKE STOPPING

Connections with concealed spaces in the walls or other areas of the building should be blocked to prevent the spread of flames. Stairways must be enclosed to protect them from fire as well as to keep them from serving as a root for flame spread. Fire doors must exist in hallways, stairs, dumbwaiters and laundry chutes to prevent the spread of superheated air, toxic gases and smoke.

231

SEGREGATION OF AREAS AND ACTIVITIES

Areas and activities inherently susceptible to fire must be segregated. Isolation within fire-resistant rooms of such operations as heating plants, storage and use of combustible materials, workshops and similar equipment and activities will prevent the spread of fire and make it more controllable.

INTERIOR CONSTRUCTION MATERIALS

Fire-resistant materials and paints, flame-resistant lumber and other finishes should be used as materials of construction. Structural members constructed of fire-resistant material may prevent collapse of the building, thereby allowing for escape or evacuation.

Equipment such as heating plants, electrical systems, appliances and similar items, when improperly installed, overloaded or used in a careless manner, may be sources of fire.

Readily combustible and highly flammable material must be kept to a minimum by prompt removal of rubbish and the use of noncombustible materials wherever practical. Every opportunity must be taken to substitute noncombustible materials where combustible materials are now used. This applies to furnishings such as beds, chairs, bedside tables and portable storage closets.

THE BUILDING OCCUPANTS

Staff. A trained staff member qualified to initiate emergency procedures must be awake and on duty at all times. In the case of fire this means notifying fire departments, evacuating patients and similar emergency activities. An attempt to merely put out the fire with extinguishers is not sufficient. Local and state fire marshals should be called upon to provide instruction and consultation to staff personnel at regularly scheduled intervals.

Smoking. Patients should not be permitted to smoke in bed unless closely supervised. Smoking rules must be established and enforced for both staff and patients as a fire safety factor. Regulated and supervised smoking periods are recommended. The use of metal or glass ash trays that do not have a lip for placing burning cigarettes may provide some measure of safety.

Housekeeping. Orderliness and established safe housekeeping procedures are vital safety factors. The development of a safety check sheet designed for use by the staff is most helpful in teaching recognition of hazards and in education of personnel in fire safety. Staff must be thoroughly trained in proper housekeeping procedures to eliminate hazards.

TRAINING

All new employees should be trained in the use of extinguishers, activation of alarms and evacuation procedures. Individuals most likely to fight fires are engineers, guards, housekeepers, nurses and laboratory personnel. A fire drill must be conducted at least once quarterly on each of the three shifts. Provisions should be made for emergency generators, lanterns and flashlights to provide light and power to critical areas such as stairwells, communications equipment, fire pumps and resuscitators. There should be first aid emergency facilities for employees.

The emergency teams should include at least 10 members of the staff, including maintenance personnel.

Coordination with public fire companies should also be included in the training program. It is preferable that a written agreement including information on plant layout and location of fire plugs and other necessary equipment be made with public fire companies. The types and quantities of portable extinguishers required for protection should be furnished and located according to local ordinances. Other sections of this manual deal with this subject.

INSPECTIONS

All types of fire inspections should be made on a schedule, including the following:

Inspections by the public fire department to orient the fire fighters to the hospital plan and to coordinate plans with the hospital emergency force.

Inspection by the safety officer of fire fighting and alerting facilities, such as the alarm system, fire extinguishers, water supply, standpipe, hose system and sprinklers.

Inspection by the safety officer to correct conditions such as trash accumulations; poor housekeeping practices; blocked or otherwise inadequate exits; open stairwell doors; paint-stuck hose cabinet doors; inadequately trained personnel; inadequate posted instructions; congested, overloaded or poorly maintained storage areas; and inadequately labeled utility controls.

Inspection by supervisors followed by safety officers — spot checks for such hazards as improper storage of flammable liquids and compressed gas cylinders; use of inadequate ash trays or none at all; steam sterilizing of cellulose nitrate tubes and explosion hazards, neglecting to turn off Bunsen burners when personnel are not present; excessive lengths, quantities and arrangements of extension cords; inadequate disposal facilities for hazardous chemicals; and no warning placards in immediate area of patients receiving oxygen therapy.

REGULATIONS

Basic rules established for fire protection and prevention are included in this manual and should be known to all employees and physicians. Specific rules which must be enforced by management are as follows:

Keep stairwell doors closed at all times.

Keep room doors and corridor doors closed.

Discard refuse promptly.

Do not discard chemicals into refuse cans.

Provide suitable ash trays.

Free any paint-stuck equipment or apertures.

Identify utility controls clearly.

Do not store equipment or materials in corridors.

Do not store flammable liquids in unsafe refrigerators.

Do not smoke while refueling office duplicating machines.

Confine work papers at night.

Learn how to use fire extinguishers.

FIRE CONTROLS

Detection

The use of automatic fire warning systems with detection stations in remote or inaccessible parts of the building can be of life-saving value in the event of fire. Should such systems be installed, regular testing schedules should be established to check their operation.

Sprinkler Systems

Sprinkler systems may be required in certain types of non–fire-resistant buildings. Sprinkler systems require surveillance by specially trained persons to insure that they are in working order at all times. An adequate water supply is also essential to their operation.

Extinguishers

There are certain areas of the extended care facility where fire extinguishers are required. Extinguishers can be most valuable, but only if the proper type is available for the particular problem at hand. A regular schedule of inspection must be made for all fire extinguishers.

PROCEDURE TO FOLLOW IN CASE OF FIRE OR HAZARDOUS SITUATION

1. Remove patients from the immediate hazard area and confine the hazard by shutting the door. If a patient is receiving oxygen, continue administration with emergency equipment.
2. Shut off oxygen in any room where fire is discovered.
3. Sound fire alarm.
4. Call all nursing and housekeeping personnel to the nurses' station by means of the intercom.
5. Send a messenger to the unit kitchen to request that nutrition personnel and other food service employees report to the nurses' station.
6. Direct emergency personnel to the emergency scene.
7. Turn on all corridor lights.
8. Request that ambulatory patients and visitors walk away from the center of the building toward the adjacent cross-corridors, unless passageway is obstructed.
9. Disconnect bell cords of bedridden patients located in the area adjacent to the immediate hazard zone, and evacuate (in bed) upon instructions from medical officer in charge. If the physician is not present the nurse in charge should evaluate the situation to determine the necessity for evacuation of a particular bed patient.
10. All seriously ill or disturbed patients who are evacuated should be attended if possible.
11. After evacuation of all patients, close room doors and all corridor doors.
12. Make certain that all patients have been removed from the unit. Check all rooms, including treatment rooms, bathrooms and so forth.
13. Instruct patients to remain in the evacuation area and away from the area adjacent to the corridor doors. Take a census of patients.

PROCEDURE IN UNITS OTHER THAN THAT
IN WHICH EMERGENCY OCCURS

1. When warning system (alarm, etc.) operates and emergency situation is announced over speaker system, all nursing, nutrition and housekeeping personnel should continue normal duties, but should review in their own minds their pre-assigned duties in the event that patient evacuation is ordered.

2. Be alert for further orders via speaker system.

3. Return to normal duty (if it has been interrupted) upon the announcement over the speaker system that the emergency has ended.

Note: During a period of emergency, do not allow use of the telephone unless it is imperative.

TABLE 19–1. SMALL FIRE-EXTINGUISHING APPARATUS

TYPE OF EXTINGUISHER	CLASS OF OF FIRE*	AGENT AND OPERATING CHARACTERISTICS
Hand pump	A	Contains plain water; 2½-gallon size lasts 50–55 seconds, discharges 30–40 feet; use on fires involving wood, paper, textiles, etc.
Soda acid	A	Contains bicarbonate of soda solution; 2½-gallon size lasts 50–55 seconds, discharges 30–40 feet; use on wood, paper, textiles, etc.; to operate, turn upside down.
Gas cartridge	A	Contains water and cartridge of carbon dioxide; 2½-gallon size lasts 50–55 seconds, discharges 30–40 feet; use on wood, paper, textiles, etc.; may also be used on small oil, grease, gasoline, or paint fires; to operate, turn over and pump.
Foam	A and B	Contains solution of aluminum sulfate and bicarbonate of soda; 2½-gallon size lasts 50–55 seconds, discharges 30–40 feet; use on oil, gasoline, grease and paint; to operate, turn upside-down.
Carbon dioxide	B	Contains liquid carbon dioxide under pressure; 15-pound size lasts about 42 seconds, discharges 6–8 feet; use on oil, gasoline, grease, and paint; to operate, pull pin and open valve.
Vaporizing liquid	C	Contains carbon tetrachloride and other chemicals; 1-quart size lasts 40–45 seconds, discharges 20–30 feet; use on live electric equipment; to operate, turn handle, then pump by hand. (Because of their extreme danger, use of carbon tetrachloride extinguishers is discouraged.)
Dry chemical	A and C	Contains bicarbonate of soda, dry chemicals and cartridge of carbon dioxide gas; 30-pound size lasts about 22–25 seconds, discharges about 14 feet; use on live electric equipment; to operate, pull pin and open valve (or press lever), then squeeze nozzle valve.

*Class A—wood, paper, excelsior and other ordinary combustible materials.
Class B—flammable liquids such as gasoline, kerosene or oil.
Class C—fire in electrical equipment, where the use of an extinguishing agent which does not conduct electricity is necessary.

CHAPTER TWENTY

BARBER AND BEAUTICIAN SERVICES

Personal appearance is an important factor in maintaining mental and physical health under any circumstances. Patients need and enjoy the services of barbers and beauticians.

To protect patients from accidents, infections and infestations, the facilities, the equipment and the methods that are employed must meet strict standards.

FACILITIES

WORKING AREA

A barbering and beauty center should be located in quarters that have been either designed or altered to accommodate these services. Such quarters must be large enough so that the operators are not hampered in their work and must be easy to keep clean and sanitary at all times.

WATER

Conveniently located hot and cold running water outlets are necessary.

LIGHT

The tools and materials that are dealt with in barbering and beauty work possess average contrast between light and dark limits; detail is moderately fine, and critical visibility is required only periodically. Glare-free light at the 30- to 50-foot-candle level is recommended.

OTHER UTILITIES

Some barbering and beauty services equipment (such as hairdryers, clippers and other small appliances) operate on either gas or electricity. Unless proper connections in ample quantity are installed in the working area, electrical circuits are likely to be overloaded by the use of makeshift arrangements. These arrangements pose fire and accident hazards. Local building codes require that all electrical equipment be grounded and that gas-operated equipment be vented. Compliance with these requirements is mandatory whether or not a code is in effect.

WASTE DISPOSAL

The means by which other facility wastes are disposed are adequate for the disposal of liquid and solid wastes from beauty and barbering operations. Any means that are less sanitary or efficient are not acceptable.

SUPPLIES

STORAGE SPACE

Clean, convenient storage is needed for supplies of freshly laundered towels. There should be enough freshly laundered towels that the same towel need never be used on more than one patron. It is completely unacceptable to dry towels or to dip used towels into a basin of hot water and then reuse them.

DISPOSAL CONTAINERS

Separate containers are needed for soiled and clean towels — and it should be ascertained that each container is used only for the type of towel for which it is intended. It is essential that single-service papers (or clean towels) be placed on temporary covers and headrests to prevent patrons' skin from touching them.

OPERATORS

HYGIENE

It is mandatory that operators wash their hands with soap and water before serving any patron and after serving each patron.

APPLICATION OF MATERIALS

Only powdered or liquid astringents, applied either with a clean, unused towel or with a single-service cotton applicator, are permissible. The use of styptic pencils, lump alum, powder puffs and sponges are invitations to the spread of infection: They cannot be tolerated.

HANDLING OF MATERIALS

The use of a spatula or similar tool is the only acceptable means of removing creams or other semisolid substances from their containers. Fingers are not to be used. Spatulas and similar tools are not to be allowed to touch a patron's skin.

STORAGE OF MATERIALS

Containers for waving solutions and for other liquids that are brought into personal contact with patrons are acceptable only if there is no way for the solution in the container to get contaminated. The same fluid is never to be used for more than one patron.

DISINFECTION AND STERILIZATION OF EQUIPMENT

Any equipment or instruments (other than neck dusters and clothing covers) that have touched the neck, face or head of a patron should be cleaned and disinfected before being used again. All other furniture, equipment, tools and utensils must also be kept clean and sanitary at all times.

There are many methods of disinfection and sterilization. Some methods employ "traditional" procedures and proprietary compounds. The effectiveness of any method used should be verified by the local governmental regulatory agency. Most states and cities have codified regulations that describe acceptable sanitation procedures for barbering and beauty culture operations. Some examples of methods recommended in regulations concerning disinfection of *cleaned* articles are:

Exposure to live steam for 12 minutes (roughly equivalent to autoclaving).

Immersion in a solution of or equal to 5 per cent carbolic acid, 70 per cent alcohol or 10 per cent commercial formalin for one minute.

Immersion in boiling water for not less than one minute.

Immersion in a 5 per cent aqueous solution of carbolic acid, 65 per cent alcohol, for not less than 10 minutes.

Immersion in liquor cresolis compositus USP solution for 15 minutes; or boiling in 10 per cent solution of liquor cresolis compositus USP for 3 minutes, or in 3.8 per cent solution of formaldehyde for 15 minutes.

Clipper blades: Immersion in a hot oil bath of proper viscosity for 2 minutes at between 194° and 212° F. The oil must have boiling point of between 302° and 482° F. and a flash point in excess of 230° F. The oil is heated by an electrical device thermostatically controlled to maintain a temperature between 199° and 212° F., the heating element of which must be enclosed and insulated from the frame of the device and must not be in contact with the liquid. In other respects the appliance must conform to the provisions of the Underwriters' Laboratories Standards for Electric Heating Appliances. The clipper blades should be agitated two or three times for periods of 5 to 10 seconds each while they are in the bath. The oil container must be cleaned at the end of each day and shall be filled with new, unused oil.

CHAPTER TWENTY-ONE

UTILIZATION REVIEW PLAN

An acceptable utilization review plan must provide for the review, on a sample or other basis, of admissions, durations of stay and professional services furnished, and a review of each case of continuous extended duration.

The review plan should have as its overall objectives the maintenance of high-quality patient care, more effective utilization of extended care services, the encouragement of appropriate utilization and the assurance of continuity of care on discharge.

The review must include study of such conditions as overuse and underuse of services, proper use of consultation, proper level of nursing and related care and a review of the length of stay of any in-patient for purposes of determining the necessity of continued stay.

RESPONSIBILITY FOR PLAN

The operation of the utilization review plan is the responsibility of the medical profession. It should include advice and consultation with all the appropriate professional personnel within the facility and with the administrator.

STATEMENT OF PLAN

The facility must have a currently applicable written description of its utilization review plan, including the organization and composition of the committee responsible for the utilization review, its frequency of meeting, the type of records to be kept, the method to be used in selecting cases, the definition of what constitutes the period or periods of extended duration, the relationship to claims administration by a third party, committee reports and the responsibility of the administrator in support of utilization review.

239

UTILIZATION REVIEW

(This section to be completed by person responsible for medical records)

1. _____
(Extended Care Facility-Name, Address, City & State, Zip Code)

2. _____ 3. _____ 4. _____ 5. _____
(PATIENT Identification Number)　(Age)　(sex)　(E.C.F. Admission Date)

6. Admitted to Extended Care Facility from: (please circle)

    a) Acute Hospital　　　　　　　　Number of Days Stay_____
    b) Home After Hospital Discharge　Number of Days Home_____
    c) Another E.C.F.　　　　　　　　Number of Days Stay_____

7. Admitting Diagnosis: (Primary) _____
   (Other)_____

8. Present Diagnosis: a) Same as admitting_____
   b) Changed to and/or additional: _____

9. Has/Is patient receiving therapy: Yes___ No___ a)Physical_____b)Speech___
   c) Number of treatments___d) Date of last treatment _____

10. Date of last visit by attending physician _____

11. Attending physician's recommendations for continued care (please summarize)
_____
_____
_____

12. Days in this E.C.F. to current date_____ Date of last review_____ Date _____

(This section to be completed by nursing supervisor.) Please circle as appropriate.)
13. Mental Status: a) alert　b) confused　c) forgetful

14. Behavior: a) cooperative　b) belligerent　c) noisy　d) senile　e) withdrawn
   f) socializes

15. Impairments: a) aphasic　b) hearing　c) speech　d) sensation　e) vision
   f) language

16. Incontinence: a) bladder　b) bowel　c) catheter

17. Care Status: a) bedridden　b) bed-chair　c) if b how long up daily
   (Please use code for items below: I-independent　A-assistance　U-unable to do)

d) ambulation	e) transfer	f) dressing
alone _____	bed-wheelchair _____	complete _____
attendent _____	wheelchair-toilet_____	upper extremities_____
cane _____	wheelchair-tub _____	trunk _____
walkerette _____		lower extremities_____
wheelchair _____		prosthesis _____
		(type) _____

UTILIZATION REVIEW — Continued

g) hygiene   h) feeding   i) diet (check one)   j) injections required:

bathing_____ fork_____ regular_____   yes_____ no_____

dental_____ spoon_____ blended_____   (circle as applies)

hair_____ knife_____ liquid_____   has been taught, could

shaving_____ glass_____ tube fed_____   be taught, cannot learn

cup_____ therapeutic_____   proper technique.

fed_____ (type)_____

Type _____

18. Patient's condition has: improved_____ deteriorated_____ remained static_____
since admission to this E.C.F. _____ since last review_____

19. _____

Signature of nurse making this report   Date of report

Space is provided on back for information of other professional personnel
if it is felt desirable to include.

(Complete in triplicate, retain one copy and send two copies to UR Committee)

20. Supplemental information from paramedical consultants; summarized:

_____

_____

_____

_____

UTILIZATION REVIEW COMMITTEE CHECK LIST
(To be completed by reviewing physician)

Check as appropriate with explanatory note if necessary:

1. Was admission to E.C.F. necessary or could services have been provided
by a home health agency or in another type facility: Yes_____ No _____
Comment: _____

2. Could lenth of stay in E.C.F. have been shortened without adverse effect
to patient?   Yes_____ No_____
Comment:_____

3. Was appropriate use made of ancillary services to shorten patient's stay
in E.C.F.?_____ Yes_____ No_____
Comment:

4. Are additional services necessary?   Yes_____ No_____
a) If YES please indicate type _____

UTILIZATION REVIEW — Continued

5. Is further stay recommended:
   If <u>YES</u> complete the following:
   a) Reason for continued stay _____
   b) Date of next review _____
   If <u>NO</u> complete the following: (U.R. Chairman see also below)*
   c) Reason discontinuation is recommended _____
   _____

   d) Recommendation for other type are (if any)_____
   _____

6. Date of review_____ Signature or code number.
   of reviewing physician. _____

7. Date _____ Signature or code number
   of the U.R.C. Chairman_____

8. TO BE COMPLETED IF CONTINUED STAY IS <u>DISAPPROVED</u>:
   Letter sent to following:
   a) attending physician_____ Date _____
   b) facility_____Date _____
   c) responsible party_____Date _____

FOR USE OF THE FACILITY ONLY

Sent to U.R.C. on _____ Returned after review on _____

Decision _____

Disposition and/or date of next review _____

CONDUCT OF REVIEW

The utilization review of the extended care facility should be conducted by a staff committee of the facility which is composed of two or more physicians, preferably with the inclusion of other professional personnel.

BASES FOR REVIEW

Reviews must be made of admissions, duration of stays and professional services, including drugs and biologicals furnished, with respect to the medical necessities of the services, for the purpose of promoting the most efficient use of available health facilities and services.

Such reviews must emphasize identification and analysis of patterns of patient care to maintain consistent high quality.

The review should be accomplished by the studies of medical records of patients of the institution.

EXTENDED DURATION CASES

The extended care facility's utilization review must specify the number of continuous days of stay in the extended care facility, following which a review must be made to determine whether further in-patient extended care services are medically necessary.

Reviews must be made no later than the seventh day following the last day of the period of extended duration specified in the plan.

No physician may review any case of continuous extended duration in which he was professionally involved. The judgment of the attending physician in an extended care stay is given great weight and is not rejected except under unusual circumstances. However, should he determine that further in-stay is not medically necessary, the physician members of the committee must request a study and consultation of the case. They must notify the attending physician within 48 hours of their evaluation. In addition, the patient or his representatives must be also notified.

MAINTENANCE OF RECORDS OF REVIEW

The administrator of the extended care facility must act upon administrative recommendations made by the utilization review committee.

Records must be kept of the activities of the committee, and reports regularly made to the administrator. A summary of the number and types of cases reviewed and the findings must be part of the records of the committee. Minutes of each committee meeting must be maintained.

Committee action in extended stay cases must be recorded with cases identified only by case number when possible.

STAFF COOPERATION WITH REVIEW COMMITTEE

An individual must be designated who is responsible for the review service. The extended care facility must make available to the attending physician current information on resources available for continued non-institutional or custodial care of patients, and must arrange for prompt transfer with appropriate medical and nursing information in order to assure continuity of care upon discharge of a patient.

You will find the appropriate committee make-up in accordance with the established procedure in Chapter 3, "Patient Care Policies."

CHAPTER TWENTY-TWO

BUSINESS SERVICES

MANAGEMENT AND ACCOUNTING

Management entails the direction of resources toward the attainment of objectives. In a health care institution such as yours, the primary objective is that of providing quality services at optimum cost, to earn a reasonable return on the owner's investment.

The aim of *controlling* is that of assuring that the objectives of an organization are realized. The main elements of a control process are comparison of

ORGANIZATION CHART

```
                              ┌──────────────────┐
                              │  Administration  │
                              └──────────────────┘
            ┌──────────────────────┼──────────────────────┐
   ┌──────────────────┐   ┌──────────────────┐   ┌──────────────────┐
   │  Daily Services  │   │ Special Services │   │ General Services │
   └──────────────────┘   └──────────────────┘   └──────────────────┘
         │                      │                      │
     ┌────────┐          ┌────────────────┐      ┌──────────────────┐
     │ Unit A │          │ Physician Care │      │ Dietary          │
     └────────┘          └────────────────┘      └──────────────────┘
     ┌────────┐          ┌────────────────┐      ┌──────────────────┐
     │ Unit B │          │ Pharmacy       │      │ Laundry and Linen│
     └────────┘          └────────────────┘      └──────────────────┘
     ┌────────┐          ┌────────────────┐      ┌──────────────────┐
     │ Unit C │          │ Laboratory     │      │ Housekeeping     │
     └────────┘          └────────────────┘      └──────────────────┘
     ┌────────┐          ┌────────────────┐      ┌──────────────────┐
     │ Unit D │          │ Radiology      │      │ Plant Operation  │
     └────────┘          └────────────────┘      └──────────────────┘
                         ┌────────────────┐      ┌──────────────────┐
                         │ Recreation     │      │ Plant Maintenance│
                         └────────────────┘      └──────────────────┘
                         ┌────────────────┐      ┌──────────────────────┐
                         │ Rehabilitation │      │ General Administration│
                         └────────────────┘      └──────────────────────┘
```

actual and planned performance, analysis of any significant deviations and corrective action.

The effectiveness of management functions of planning and control depends largely upon the soundness of the organizational structure; the adequacy of financial and statistical data relating to each unit within the institution; and the ability of management to make intelligent use of such data. Accounting, therefore, is a vital and integral part of the management process.

ACCOUNTING CONVENTIONS

In order to give the necessary completeness, accuracy and meaningfulness to accounting data, the accrual basis of accounting should be employed by the health care institution. This system gives accounting recognition to revenues earned in the time period and to expenses incurred in the time period regardless of the flow of cash. Accrued income is income that has been earned but not yet received in cash. For example, at the end of a week the services rendered to a patient may not have been paid yet, but they have been earned by the institution.

Conversely, accrued expense is expense that has been incurred by the institution but not yet paid in cash. An example is salaries and wages earned by employees during the work period but not yet paid.

REVENUE

Revenue consists mainly of the value of all services rendered to patients regardless of the amount actually paid to the institution. This revenue should be accumulated in the accounts in a manner that identifies the revenue with the organizational units that produced the revenue. Measurement of patient service revenue can then be compared with direct expenses in those units so that the performance of each organizational unit can be planned and controlled more effectively.

EXPENSES

Expenses are costs that have been incurred in carrying on the operating activities of the organization. Complete and meaningful records of expenses must be recorded in a manner which clearly associates them with the responsible organizational unit within the institution.

MATCHING REVENUES AND EXPENSES

Determination of the net income for an accounting period, then, requires the measurement of amounts of revenue or revenue deductions and of expenses that are associated with that period. Revenue must be recorded in the period in which it is earned, and measurement must be made of expenses incurred in rendering the services on which the revenue determination was based. Unless there is a matching of accomplished revenue and expense within each accrual period, the reported net income for the period is meaningless.

THE ACCOUNTING PROCESS

Accounting is described as the accumulation and communication of quantitative data relating to the activities of an organization and the interpretation of the results of such data. Accumulation is the mechanical process of making records of financial transactions. Communication is the reporting of such information to management and other users of financial and statistical data.

Following is a description of the procedures to be followed in keeping records of transactions.

THE ACCOUNTING SYSTEM

An accounting system includes a chart of accounts, documentary evidence of transactions, a journal and a ledger.

CHART OF ACCOUNTS

The manner in which transactions are to be classified in accounting is indicated by what is known as a chart of accounts. This is designed to provide the framework for a systematic accumulation of financial data in groupings that will meet legal, tax and regulatory agency requirements. A simplified chart of accounts follows:

No. 100 Assets
     101 Cash
     102 Accounts receivable
     103 Inventory
     104 Prepaid insurance
     150 Land
     151 Building
     152 Accumulated depreciation – building
     153 Equipment
     154 Accumulated depreciation – equipment
No. 200 Liabilities
     201 Accounts payable
     202 Salaries and wages payable
     203 Mortgage payable
No. 300 Capital
     301 Owner, capital
     302 Owner, drawings
     303 Revenue and expense summary
No. 400 Revenue
     401 Daily service
     402 Special service
No. 500 Expenses
     501 Salaries and wages
     502 Supplies

503 Utilities and telephone
504 Advertising
505 Repairs
506 Depreciation
507 Insurance
508 Interest

Each account in the chart is assigned an identifying number to save clerical time and work. It is easier, for example, to write "501" than it is to write "Salaries and wages expense."

Assets

Assets are things of value owned by the institution. Account 101, cash, for example, represents the amount of money on deposit in the bank. Account 102, accounts receivable, reflects the amount due from patients for services rendered to them. Account 103, inventory, carries the cost of unused supplies on hand. Account 104, prepaid insurance, shows the amount of insurance premiums paid in advance.

Accounts also provide for the value of land, buildings and equipment owned by the institution.

Accounts 152 and 154, accumulated depreciation, show the portion of the cost of buildings and equipment that have been depreciated, that is charged to expense.

Liabilities

Liabilities are the debts of the institution.

Account 201, accounts payable, represents the amount owed to creditors for supplies and services purchased by the institution.

Account 202, salaries and wages payable, reflects the amount of salaries and wages earned by the employees but not yet paid to them.

Account 203, mortgage payable, shows the amount owed to a bank on a mortgage.

Capital

Capital is the equity of the owner in the institution; that is, the amount of the owner's investment.

A drawings account is provided to record the amount withdrawn from the institution by the owner for his own personal use.

Revenues

Account 401, daily service revenue, is used to record the revenues earned from rendering daily service, room, board, and general nursing care to patients.

Accounts 402, special service revenue, shows the revenue derived from special services such as pharmacy, laboratory, radiology, physical therapy and others.

Expenses

The chart of accounts provides accounts for recording expenses in eight classifications: salaries and wages; supplies; utilities and telephone; advertising; repairs; depreciation; insurance; and interest.

DOCUMENTARY EVIDENCE

Competent documentary evidence of completed transactions is a fundamental requirement. Purchase orders, invoices, vouchers, checks, cash receipt slips and other documents give evidence of completed transactions and provide information needed to record the transactions.

THE JOURNAL

The journal is a business diary in which a written chronological record of business transactions is made. The general journal consists of formal analyses of the increase and decrease effects of transactions on the assets, liabilities, capital, revenue and expenses of the institution. The general journal is divided as follows (see p. 252):

The first column on the left records the date on which the transaction occurred. Often, transactions of the same type—charges to patients for services, for example—may be summarized weekly, bi-weekly or monthly instead of daily. In such cases the summary entry is dated the day it is entered in the journal.

The second column from the left, entitled accounts and explanations, is for recording the names of the accounts increased or decreased by the transaction. Also in this column, the transaction is briefly described. The title of the account debited is written first, against the left-hand margin of the column. The title of the account credited is written underneath the name of the account debited and is indented. This is done to distinguish the credits from the debits at a glance. The description of the transaction should be further indented to distinguish it from the title of the account credited.

The third column is the account number column. The numbers of the accounts debited and credited are entered in these columns.

The last two columns are, in order, "Debit" and "Credit." The dollar amounts involved in a transaction are written in the debit and credit columns as indicated.

A line should be skipped between journal entries so that each entry is set apart from the others on the same journal page.

Debits and Credits

The word debit simply refers to the left-hand side of an accounting record—the left-hand money column in a journal, for example—and the word credit refers to the right-hand side. Entries are made on the left and right sides of accounting records to record the increase and decrease effects of transactions on the accounts listed in the chart of accounts. For example, increases in asset and expense accounts are assigned to the debit side. Decreases in these accounts are recorded by making credit (right-hand) entries. The rule is reversed for liability, capital and revenue accounts: decreases in liability, capital and revenue are assigned to the debit side, and increases are assigned to the credit side.

Every journal entry will include at least one debit and one credit, and the debits and credits in any journal entry must be equal in amount. This equality keeps the books in balance.

Example: The institution purchased supplies on February 2 at a cost of $1,450. This transaction would be recorded in the general journal as follows:

Under the date: February 2.

Under accounts and explanations: Supplies expense, Account No. 502. (You will note in the chart of accounts that 500 indicates expenses; 502, under the major heading of 500, is for supplies.)

In the debit column, the cost: $1450.00.

In the accounts and explanations column an item listed as accounts payable must be recorded to indicate an expense.

The debit column already carries the value (cost) of the supplies as an asset.

The credit column should now contain the same figure, $1450.00 to indicate that an expense has been incurred.

Under account number, 201 should be recorded. (200 is for liabilities, 201 is for accounts payable.

In the accounts and explanation column, beneath the account titles of accounts payable and supplies expense, should be recorded a brief description of the purchase. For example: Purchase of supplies on account from General Supply Company.

The recording of this transaction is now complete. The next entry into the general journal is separated from this one by skipping a line, and the identical procedure is again followed.

THE LEDGER

The general journal provides a chronological record of the effects of total transactions on the accounts used by the institution. It does not, however, reflect account balances, which are needed in order to prepare financial statements at the end of the month. To determine the balances of the various accounts at the end of the month, the information recorded in the general journal is transferred to individual ledger accounts. Such a ledger account is maintained for each account in the chart of accounts. (See p. 253.) The transfer of recorded information from the general journal to the individual ledger accounts is called "posting." The following points should be noted about journals and ledgers.

A separate ledger page is maintained for each account listed in the chart of accounts. Together, all the accounts are referred to as a general ledger. This often consists of many pages.

No entry can be made in a ledger account until an entry has been made in the journal. The journal is the book of original entry; the ledger is the book of secondary entry. In other words, the general journal shows every single transaction that has been made, whereas a ledger account shows only those transactions that apply to a particular account, such as accounts payable. All of the accounts payable, appearing in many and varied locations within the general journal, are summarized in the ledger account titled "Accounts Payable" one after the other.

Each ledger page indicates an account title and the number of that account as shown in the chart of accounts.

The date of the journal entry being posted (that is, the transaction date that was originally entered into the general journal) is copied into the column on the left side of the ledger page.

The reference column of the ledger page is used to indicate the page number of the journal on which the posted entry appears. By indicating account numbers in the journal (in the accounts and explanations column), and journal page numbers in the ledger, a cross-index for locating specific data is established.

The amount of the debit or credit recorded in the journal is written into the debit or credit column of the ledger form.

The balance of the ledger account after each posting is indicated in the balance column.

The narrow column on the far right of the ledger page is used to indicate whether the balance of the account is a debit balance or a credit balance. Asset and expense accounts normally have debit balances. Other accounts usually have credit balances.

Work Sheet

After all transactions for a month have been journalized and posted, and month-end balances have been determined in each ledger account, a work sheet should be prepared. (See p. 259.) The steps in preparation of a work sheet are as follows:

List the accounts in the general ledger with their month-end balances extended into the unadjusted trial balance column of the work sheet.

Enter any adjusting entries that are required in the adjustment section of the work sheet.

Extend the adjusted figures into the adjusted trial balance columns.

Extend the adjusted trial balance figures into the appropriate financial statement columns. Debit balances in the adjusted trial balance are extended as debits. Credit balances are extended as credits.

Add the debit and credit columns of the income statement section. The difference between these totals is the income for the period and is extended into the capital statement section as a credit. In case of a net loss, the net loss would appear as a balancing credit in the income statement section and would be extended into the capital statement section as a debit.

Add the debit and credit columns of the capital statement section. The difference between these totals is the amount of the owner's capital on a particular date. This figure is extended into the balance sheet section as a credit.

Add the debit and credit columns of the balance sheet section to ascertain that the accounts are in balance.

Financial Statement

An income statement, a statement of owner's capital and a balance sheet may now be prepared directly from the information shown on the work sheet. (See pp. 253 and 254.)

Income statement

An income statement, also referred to as a profit and loss statement or a statement of income and expense, reflects the results of operations in terms of revenue earned and expenses incurred. (See p. 253.)

Statement of owner's equity

A statement of owner's equity shows the changes that have occurred in the amount of the owner's equity during a given period of time. This statement is also called a statement of retained earnings. (See p. 253.)

Balance sheet

The balance sheet reflects the financial position of the institution in terms of its assets, liabilities and capital at a given date. (See p. 254.)

Adjusting entries

The next step in the accounting cycle is to journalize and post the adjusting entries which appear on the work sheet. When this is completed the general ledger will contain the same balances as shown in the adjusted trial balance section of the work sheet. Monthly adjusting entries should be entered on the work sheet only, and should not be journalized and posted to the general ledger. Financial statements are prepared directly from the adjusted trial balance figures shown on the work sheet. This practice simplifies the preparation of monthly accounting reports.

Closing the books

The process described in the preceding sections continues month after month during the fiscal year. At the end of the fiscal year, however, an additional procedure is necessary. The balances of revenue and expense accounts must be removed from the general ledger. This is known as closing the books. It is done annually so that the net income or net loss for each year can more easily be determined. The annual closing is accomplished by journalizing and posting the closing entries. In other words, entries are made in a journal which, after they are posted, will eliminate the revenue and expense account balances and the drawings account balance from the general ledger. The procedure for closing the books is as follows:

Debit all revenue accounts individually in the amount of their balances and credit the total to the revenue and expense summary account. The revenue accounts are debited because they have credit balances.

Credit all expense accounts individually in the amount of their balances and debit the total to the revenue and expense summary account. The expense accounts are credited because they have debit balances.

Close the balance of the revenue and expense summary account to the owner's capital account: Where the operations have produced a net income, debit the amount of net income to the revenue and expense summary account and credit the owner's capital account. Where operations have produced a net loss, credit the amount of net loss to the revenue and expense summary account and debit the owner's capital account.

Debit the owner's capital account and credit the owner's drawings account for the amount of the owner's drawings for the year.

When these entries have been posted the general ledger will contain only the year-end balance sheet accounts. These balances are carried over into the next fiscal year and a new accounting cycle begins.

GENERAL JOURNAL

19-- Date		Accounts and Explanations	Acct. No.	Debit	Credit

LEDGER ACCOUNT

ACCOUNT TITLE				ACCOUNT NO.			

19-- Date			Ref.	Debit	Credit	Balance	Dr. Cr.

INCOME STATEMENT

Period Ended_____ 19____

Revenues
  Daily Service Revenues...
  Special Service Revenues..................................... _____
Total Revenues.. _____

Expenses
  Salaries and Wages...
  Supplies...
  Utilities and Telephone ....
  Advertising...
  Repairs...
  Depreciation...
  Insurance ....
  Interest .... _____
Total Expenses... _____
Net Income .... _____
                                                                              _____

STATEMENT OF OWNER'S EQUITY

Period Ended_____ 19____

Owner, Capital, January 1, 19____ ....
Add Net Income for Two Months Ended February 28, 19____................. _____
Total...
Less Drawings for Two Months Ended February 28, 19____ .... _____
Owner, Capital, February 28, 19____ .... _____

BALANCE SHEET

As of_____ 19____

ASSETS

Current Assets
    Cash ....
    Accounts Receivable ....
    Inventory ....
    Prepaid Insurance ....   _____
Total Current Assets ....   _____

Noncurrent Assets
    Land ....
    Building...
    Less Accumulated Depreciation.........   _____
    Equipment ....
    Less Accumulated Depreciation.........   _____   _____
Total Noncurrent Assets.........................   _____
Total Assets ....   ══════

LIABILITIES AND CAPITAL

Current Liabilities
    Accounts Payable ....
    Salaries and Wages Payable...............   _____
Total Current Liabilities ....
Mortgage Payable..................................   _____
Total Liabilities ....
Owner, Capital.....................................   _____
Total Liabilities and Capital ....   ══════

PATIENT'S LEDGER CARD

			Patient		Room No.	Mo. Rate	From _____

Date	Daily Service	Pharmacy	Physical Therapy	Other Description	Amount	Total
Balance, beginning of Month						
Total						
Payment received--Third Party						
Payment received--Other						

BALANCE DUE (Third Party $_____ Other $ _____)

To _____

_____

_____

SAMPLE CHARGE TICKET

CHARGE TICKET

Patient _____   Date _____

Room No. _____

Check Department

☐ Physician Care

☐ Pharmacy

☐ Laboratory

☐ Recreation

☐ Rehabilitation

☐ Special Care

Description	Charge

Total _____

Signed _____

SAMPLE CASH RECEIPT SLIP

```
Cash Receipt Slip


                                    Date _____

   Received From _____   $_____

   _____   Dollars

   For _____
   .
                       Signed _____
```

PAYROLL AND TAXES

TIME AND EARNINGS RECORDS

It is assumed that the pay period will be bi-weekly. At the first of the pay period, the employee's name and the date of the pay period are typed on a time and earnings record. The record is then given to the employee or to the employee's supervisor. At the end of each day the employee or the supervisor enters the number of hours the employee worked. At the end of the pay period the record is returned to the accounting office, where the hours worked are calculated and gross pay and deductions are entered. Finally, the record should be approved by the individual responsible.

PAYROLL JOURNAL

Employee time and earnings records serve as the basis for entries in the payroll journal. It is strongly suggested that there be two types of checking accounts maintained by the institution, one called a "general checking account" and the other a "payroll checking account."

Once the payroll for the period is determined from the payroll journal a single check for the total net payroll should be written on the general checking account and deposited in the payroll checking account. When the payroll checks clear the bank, the payroll checking account will have no balance. The bank should be instructed to charge the general checking account for the service charges of the payroll checking account. The two types of checks should be of different colors.

PAYROLL TAXES

Federal Income Tax

Federal law requires employers to make income tax withholdings from employees' salaries and wages and to remit such withholdings to the Internal

Revenue Service. The deduction to be made is determined from withholding tables furnished by the government. Use of the tables requires a knowledge of the number of exemptions claimed by each employee as indicated on Form W-4 (Employee's Withholding Exemption Certificate), which each employee must fill out.

FICA Taxes

Employers also must withhold FICA (Federal Insurance Contributions Act) tax from employees' wages. The amount to be withheld is a percentage (up to a

TIME AND EARNINGS RECORD

EMPLOYEE TIME AND EARNINGS RECORD

Employee _____ Two Weeks Ended _____

Day	DEPARTMENTAL HOURS						
	Dietary	Laundry	Housekeeping				Total Hours
Totals							
Hourly Rate							
Gross Pay							
Debit							

SUMMARY

Debit_____   _____
Debit_____   _____
Debit_____   _____
Debit_____   _____
Debit_____   _____
Gross Pay   _____
Payroll Deductions
  FICA   _____
  Income Tax   _____
Total Payroll Deductions   _____

Net Pay   _____

Check number_____

Approved_____

specified limit) of wages paid. Again the federal government provides information to all employers in regard to percentages and rates. It should be noted that the employer must match the amount paid to the government by the employee.

FUTA Taxes

Federal Unemployment Taxes are paid only by the employer. The amount of tax is a percentage (to a specified limit) of wages paid. Payments made by the employer into a state unemployment tax fund may be credited against the Federal Unemployment Tax.

PAYROLL JOURNAL

Two Weeks Ended / Employee Name	Gross Pay	Taxes Withheld		Net Pay	Check No.
		Income	FICA		

GRAND TOTAL

Credit A/C Number

WORK SHEET

	Trial Balance		Adjustments		Adjusted Trial Balance		Income Statement		Capital Statement		Balance Sheet	
	Dr.	Cr.	Dr.	Cr.	Dr.	Cr.	Dr.	Cr.	Dr.	Cr.	Dr.	Cr.
Cash												
Accounts Receivable												
Inventory												
Prepaid Insurance												
Land												
Building												
Accumulated Depreciation												
Equipment												
Accumulated Depreciation												
Accounts Payable												
Salaries and Wages Payable												
Mortgage Payable												
Owner, Capital												
Owner, Drawings												
Daily Service Revenue												
Special Service Revenue												
Salaries and Wages Expense												
Supplies Expense												
Utilities and Telephone Expense												
Advertising Expense												
Repairs Expense												
Depreciation Expense												
Insurance Expense												
Interest Expense												
Totals												
Net Income												
Totals												
Owner, Capital												
Totals												

ACCOUNTING CYCLE SUMMARY

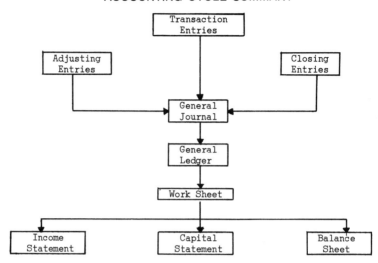

Remittance of Payroll Taxes

Each month (except April, July, October and January) the institution must remit through a local commercial bank, using Form 450, Federal Depository Receipt, the total of (1) employees' and employer's FICA taxes and (2) federal income taxes withheld on the preceding month's payroll. (For these taxes, the institution must file Form 941 on or before the last day of the first month following each calendar quarter.)

On this return, each employee's FICA number, name and taxable wages received during the quarter must be reported. The FICA tax and Federal Income Tax withheld must also be indicated. Credit is taken for amounts paid on depository receipts and the balance of the tax is remitted with the return. Federal unemployment taxes are paid once each year on January 31, when form 940 is filed with the district director of the Internal Revenue Service.

REIMBURSEMENT FOR PROVIDING SERVICES UNDER TITLE XVIII

BASIS OF REIMBURSEMENT

The Medicare law directs that payments to providers of services, such as hospitals and extended care facilities, be made on the basis of the *reasonable cost* of each provider rendering services to program beneficiaries. Reasonable cost means the actual cost of providing patient care except where such costs are determined to be excessive when compared to the costs of similar institutions. It is the intent of the Medicare law that payments to providers of service should be fair to the providers and to the contributors of the health insurance trust funds and other patients.

ALLOWABLE COSTS

The principles of reimbursement essentially recognize all necessary and proper operating expenses, including salaries of necessary personnel, administrative expenses, a reasonable allowance of compensation for the services of owners performed in a necessary function, maintenance costs and interest expense. Proprietary institutions are permitted a return on equity capital invested and used in the provision of patient care. The rate of return allowable is one and one-half times the average interest rate on public debt obligations issued to the Federal Hospital Insurance Trust Fund. For purposes of computing equity capital, we generally mean a provider's net investment in all assets related to patient care, such as net working capital maintained for necessary patient care activities and net investment in plant, property, equipment and such; in other words, net of any depreciation *and* related indebtedness such as a mortgage.

Cost Apportionment Method

The items enumerated above are includable in the provider's total *allowable costs*, which must then be apportioned among the users of the facility. The reimbursement regulations establish two basic methods of apportionment, either of which may be used at the option of the provider, for determining the program's share of the provider's allowable costs. The first method is the "departmental method," which involves a relationship of Medicare charges to total patient charges applied to costs. Under this method a percentage representing the beneficiaries' share of total charges, on a department basis, is applied to total allowable costs for the respective departments. This department-by-department method involves a determination, by cost-finding methods, of the total costs for each of the institution's departments that are revenue-producing, i.e., departments providing services for which charges are made to patients. The costs of each department are then apportioned among the users of the department.

The second method is the "combination method." Under this method, the cost of routine services (room, board, nursing service) is apportioned on the basis of patient days for beneficiaries and for other patients; in other words, an average cost per inpatient day. The costs of ancillary services (such as radiology, laboratory, drugs, etc.) are apportioned on the basis of a percentage representing the beneficiaries' share of the provider's *total* charges for ancillary services. The amounts determined to be the program's share of the two parts of the provider's allowable costs are then added together to determine the total amount of reimbursement. The combination method also requires that the costs of routine services be separated from the costs of ancillary services by cost-finding methods.

Cost-Finding Method

This method recognizes that services rendered by non–revenue-producing departments or cost centers are utilized by other non–revenue-producing departments as well as by the revenue-producing departments. All costs of non–revenue-producing departments are allocated to all departments which they serve, regardless of whether or not these departments produce revenue. The costs of those departments that provide the most service and receive the least should be allocated first. After the cost of each non–revenue-producing center is allocated, that center will be considered "closed" and no further costs will be allocated to it. This applies even though it may have received some services from a center whose cost is apportioned later.

PAYMENT PROCEDURES

The Medicare program has a comprehensive payment system designed to reimburse providers of service currently so that they are not disadvantaged. Basically, providers are reimbursed on an interim basis throughout the year based on billings for services rendered. When total costs are determined at the end of the year a final settlement will be made. However, in addition to the basic payment procedure, a current financing payment can also be made *upon* the *request* of the provider. This payment is designed to reimburse providers currently as services are actually rendered to beneficiaries, and it enhances a provider's working capital position.

The primary factor in adopting an accounting system for Medicare purposes is that essential financial and statistical data must be available. The method of accounting used is left to the discretion of the institution. The Social Security Administration requires that a standard cost report indicating general categories of costs, such as nursing, dietary, operation of plant and depreciation, be used.

The owner should understand that the term reasonable cost means the actual cost of providing covered services to beneficiaries *except* where an institution's costs are *substantially out of line* with those of institutions similar in size, scope of services, utilization and other relevant factors. Actual cost will include both direct and indirect costs as well as normal standby costs. The remittance received will be equal to the actual costs determined under the principles of reimbursement in the particular institution, not an average rate for all institutions.

The principles of reimbursement provide for a reasonable allowance of compensation for services of an owner to be included as an allowable cost, provided those are actually performed in a "necessary function." A *reasonable* allowance would be governed, in part, by the amount paid for comparable services by comparable institutions under comparable circumstances. By necessary function is meant that service which the institution would ordinarily have a person other than the owner performing. The owner's salary for his services will be included in total costs and apportioned as all other costs.

The following illustrations of the methods used by a theoretical nursing home are included to aid in both determining the method best suited to your facility and understanding the procedures.

TABLE 22–1. ILLUSTRATION OF COST REIMBURSEMENT METHODS

BASIC STATISTICAL DATA

1. 110 Bed ECF

2. a. Available Bed Days — 40,150
   b. Actual Bed Days — 38,000
   c. Medicare Bed Days — 11,400 (30%)

3. Average Charge Per Day
   a. Routine Charges — $15.00
   b. Total Charges — $19.08

4. Average Cost Per Day
   a. Routine Services — $13.42
      (510,000 + 38,000)
   b. Total Costs — $16.58
      (630,000 + 38,000)

DEPARTMENT SPECIAL SERVICES	CHARGES TO PROGRAM	TOTAL CHARGES	% RATIO	TOTAL COST*	DEPARTMENTAL METHOD COST OF BENEFICIARY SERVICES
Pharmacy	$ 25,500	$ 60,000	42.5%	$ 40,000	$ 17,000
Laboratory	10,000	34,000	34.0%	25,000	8,500
X-ray	3,000	6,000	50.0%	4,000	2,000
Physical Therapy	9,000	15,000	60.0%	16,000	9,600
Speech Therapy	1,000	10,000	10.0%	8,000	800
Occupational Therapy	500	5,000	10.0%	4,000	400
Other	12,500	25,000	50.0%	23,000	11,500
Subtotal Spec. Serv.	61,500	155,000	39.7%	120,000	
Routine Services	199,500	570,000	35.0%	510,000	178,500
Total	$261,000	$725,000	36.0%	$630,000	$228,300

COMPARISON OF METHODS

METHOD	COST REIMBURSEMENT	AV. COST PER MEDICARE DAY
Departmental	$228,300	20.02
Combination	200,640	17.60
Av. Cost (16.58 × 11,400) = 189,012		16.58

COMBINATION METHOD

Gross % ratio × cost
39.7% × $120,000 = $ 47,640
Av. cost per day × Med. bed days
13.42 × 11,400 = 153,000
$200,640

*As determined by cost-finding techniques (see Table 22–2: step down method).

TABLE 22-2. STEP DOWN COST-FINDING

	DEPR.*	GEN. ADMIN.	PLANT OPERATION	DIETARY	LAUNDRY & LINEN	HOUSE-KEEPING	NURSING	MEDICAL SUPPLIES	TOTAL
GENERAL SERVICE DEPTS.									
Depr.	65,000								
Interest	12,000								
Owner's Sal.	11,000								
Specific Allow. (1½%)	9,100								
Admin.	81,700								
Total Admin.	113,800	115,100							
Plant Operation	20,000	1,000	22,100						
Dietary	80,000	3,000	1,700	86,000					
Laundry & Linen	11,000	500	1,000		14,000				
Housekeeping	34,000	500	100		100	35,000			
Nursing	200,000	13,200	800		3,000	2,000	220,000		
Medical Supplies	25,000	500	200		100	200		27,000	
SPECIAL SERVICE DEPTS.									
Routine Services	–0–	86,500	15,800	86,000	9,700	29,000	220,000	13,000	510,000
Pharmacy	30,000	5,000	1,000		300	1,700			40,000
Laboratory	20,000	1,500	500		200	800			25,000
X-ray	2,500	200	100		100	100			4,000
Physical Therapy	12,000	1,500	500		200	300			16,000
Speech Therapy	6,500	500	200		200	100			8,000
Occupational Therapy	3,200	200	100		100	200			4,000
Other	7,000	1,000	100		–	600		14,000	23,000
TOTAL	630,000								630,000

*See Table 22–3 for basis and how distribution was made.

TABLE 22–3. COMPUTATION AND DISTRIBUTION OF DEPRECIATION FOR STEP DOWN COST-FINDING

DEPARTMENT	BUILDING COST: $500,000 SQUARE FEET: 125,000		EQUIPMENT & FIXTURES TOTAL COST: $150,000			TOTAL DEPRECIATION PER STEP DOWN W/S
	% OF SQ. FT.	DEPR. AMT.	% OF COST	COST BY DEPT.	DEPR. AMT.	
Administration	2.0	1,000	2.0	3,000	300	1,300
Plant	1.0	500	4.0	6,000	600	1,100
Dietary	2.45	1,225	.5	750	75	1,300
Laundry & Linen	2.4	1,200	2.0	3,000	300	1,500
Housekeeping	.15	75	1.5	2,250	225	300
Nursing	1.4	700	2.0	3,000	300	1,000
Medical Supplies	.8	400	4.0	6,000	600	1,000
Routine Service		40,700		93,000	9,300	50,000
Pharmacy	2.2	1,100	6.0	9,000	900	2,000
Laboratory	2.8	1,400	4.0	6,000	600	2,000
X-ray	.35	175	5.5	8,250	825	1,000
Physical Therapy	2.1	1,050	3.0	4,500	450	1,500
Speech Therapy	.4	200	2.0	3,000	300	500
Occupational Therapy	.1	50	1.0	1,500	150	200
Other	.45	225	.5	750	75	300
	100.0%	$50,000	100.0%	150,000	$15,000	$65,000

CHAPTER TWENTY-THREE

ACCREDITATION

The Joint Commission on Accreditation of Hospitals, which has representation from the American Hospital Association, the American Medical Association, the American College of Physicians, the American College of Surgeons and the American Nursing Home Association, is the body responsible for surveying hospitals and nursing homes and for their certification by meeting the standards of accreditation set up by the commission. These standards are clearly written in all areas of operation of the facility and clearly define the minimum standards acceptable for certification. A survey from the commission, while voluntary in nature, carries with it automatic approval for third party payment and Medicare and Medicaid authorization from the federal government. Lack of certification places upon the facility the requirement that it be examined by the federal government (if Medicare and Medicaid services are requested) to determine its adequacy in meeting minimum standards of operation.

The following may be used as a guide or self-survey for the hospital or nursing home to determine its adequacy in connection with these minimum standards.

STATE AND LOCAL LAWS

The facility must comply with all state and local laws regarding licensure. All registered and licensed practical nurses must be licensed in the state in which they practice their profession. The facility must conform with other laws applicable, including plumbing codes, electrical codes and the like.

GOVERNING AUTHORITY

A clear definition of ownership of the facility must be declared and indications that the governing body or board of governors is the authority responsible in the operation of the facility. The governing authority must show evidence of regular meetings which describe positions and policies as to operation of the facility

ADMINISTRATION

The governing board is required to appoint an administrator who, by training and experience, is acceptable to the commission. The board must designate the administrative authority to the administrator, whose responsibilities should be clearly defined. A secondary administrative authority must be appointed to function in the absence of the administrator.

PERSONNEL

A personnel file must be kept on all employees of the facility.

All classifications must have job descriptions.

Evidence of a program of health examination and care must be available.

Authentication of licensure must be included in the files of those personnel requiring licensure.

An employment application form containing the name of next of kin for notification in the event of emergency must be included.

PATIENT CARE POLICIES

A written record of patient care policies is essential. These policies must be reviewed by the patient care policy committee annually and should cover the following areas.

Admissions
Discharges
Transfers
Physicians' services
Nursing services
Dietary services
Restorative services—physical and occupational therapy
Pharmaceutical services
Dental services
Social services
Medical records
Transfer agreements
Utilization review plans
Special care and patient activities

PHYSICIANS' SERVICES

Each patient should be admitted only on the authority of a referring physician. Prior to admission, an admission impression or diagnosis must be made. Upon admission, an admission history and physical examination must be completed.

A program of patient care must be recorded.

All physicians' orders must be written and signed.

The referring physician must take a history and perform a physical examination on admission and must visit the patient regularly after admission, in no case more rarely than weekly.

A full discharge summary must be completed prior to the discharge of the patient outlining the total care given to the patient during the period of hospitalization.

The administrative physician must be available to provide care in the event of emergency or during the absence of the attending physician.

Coverage for the administrative physician must be available and must be clearly posted with the names and telephone numbers of physicians covering the administrative physician.

NURSING

A full time director of nurses must be appointed, with the minimum qualification of nurse registration in the state.

A nursing procedure manual must be established, maintained and utilized.

Patient care policies must be available and in conformity with standards.

In-service training must be provided for all personnel.

A nursing care plan must be organized and effected for each patient.

Daily rounds of patients must be made by a registered nurse.

The medical record must reflect, in the doctors' orders, in the progress notes and in the nurses' notes, a full description of the care provided to patients.

PATIENT SUPERVISION

Nursing service must provide 24 hour nursing service to all patients.

A proper ratio of nursing personnel to patients must be maintained.

Nursing services provided to all patients by various levels of nursing personnel must be consistent with the qualification of those nursing personnel providing the care.

NURSING PLAN

The nursing care plan must respond to the needs of the patients.

The plan must be available for all nursing personnel.

The plan must be reviewed regularly and altered to suit changes in needs.

IN-SERVICE EDUCATION

All nursing personnel must be provided with an opportunity to obtain in-service education on a continuing basis.

Education opportunities must be made available to members of the nursing staff and must include training in the treatment of particular conditions of patients such as emotional disturbances and social problems.

DIETETICS

A diet formulary which includes regular and special diets is essential.

A program of assistance in patient feedings must be available.

Dietary consultation must be available for all patients and notations regarding diet therapy must be recorded in the medical record.

DIETARY SERVICES

A consultant dietitian, a member of the American Dietetic Association, must be available for consultation with administration, nursing and patients.

In-service training must be available for all dietary staff.

The quality and quantity of dietary personnel must be such that the space of time between the morning and evening meal does not exceed 14 hours.

All requirements of the local and state health departments regarding examination and certification of dietary personnel must be met.

A diet manual is essential.

A program of reporting intake and output of foods must be available.

Therapeutic diets must be clearly defined and dietary personnel made aware of their necessity.

Snacks should be available during the hours between meals and should consist of nourishing and palatable foods and beverage.

Written menus should be drawn up and posted in advance.

Adequate storage of foods must be available to provide food service for one week in the event of emergency.

Proper preparation and serving of meals is essential.

Sanitation in the main kitchen and other dietary areas of the facility must be assured.

Proper dishwashing techniques, equipment and controls, including water temperature, is required.

Proper handwashing facilities must be readily available.

Procedures of collection and discarding of unused foods must be clearly defined and adhered to.

All non-food items, including cleaning supplies, must be stored away from the area of food stuffs.

Sanitary refrigeration must be provided for ice cubes.

Regular laboratory examination for bacteria must be provided for various areas of the dietary system.

RESTORATIVE PATIENT CARE

Physical and occupational therapy consultants, certified by training and experience, must be available to those patients requiring restorative care.

All physical and occupational therapy treatments must be given on physicians' written orders only.

Only recognized nursing techniques may be used and all must be noted in the medical record.

All treatments of physical and occupational therapy must be given only under the direction of a certified therapist.

The consultant therapist should take part in planning and programing for therapy in conjunction with the medical and nursing care plans.

PHARMACY PROCEDURES

The pharmacy and therapeutics committee should develop in conjunction with the consultant pharmacist therapeutic policies, procedures and methods to be used in dispensing drugs and medicines.

The consultant pharmacist is responsible for assuring that all drugs and medicines received and dispensed to the nurses' stations be listed in the Pharmacopeia and be labeled properly with all necessary information.

The consultant pharmacist should also make an emergency kit available on all nurses' stations. The use of drugs out of the emergency kits by nursing personnel at the nurses' stations must be done only under the orders of a physician. Each of the drugs in the emergency kit must be listed on the outside of the kit, showing quantity, quality and description.

Only registered and licensed practical nurses may administer drugs and medicines to patients.

There must be a written "stop order" program for all drugs and medicines.

No more than a 24 hour supply of any drug or medicine may be given to the patient upon discharge.

All nurses' stations should have a medical reference text.

Medicine cabinets should be locked.

Narcotics cabinets should be located within the medicine cabinet, also locked.

Medicines requiring refrigeration should be kept in a biological refrigerator, not used for any other purpose other than the drugs and medicines for the nurses' stations.

All poisons should be kept under separate lock and key.

All medicines and drugs should be reviewed at intervals no greater than monthly; obsolete drugs should be discontinued, and expired drugs should be removed and destroyed by the pharmacist.

Narcotics records must be accurately kept and properly signed.

No medicines may be stored in any patients' rooms.

DIAGNOSTIC SERVICES

There must be a written policy regarding diagnostic services and a report filed in the patient's chart.

DENTAL SERVICES

A dental examination sheet should be entered in each patient's medical record, and a complete examination and recommendation should be made in writing by the consultant dentist.

SOCIAL SERVICES

There must be a consultant social worker, preferably one with a graduate advanced degree in medical social work and certified by the Society of Social Workers.

A complete record of social information should be obtained and recorded in each patient's record on admission.

Continuing social services should be available to patients and information derived therein entered in the medical record.

A consultant social worker should take part in all in-service training programs for all personnel.

All social service information must be kept confidential.

The charge nurses should be consulted by the consultant social worker in regard to the needs of each patient and records maintained on all social services entered in the patient's medical record.

PATIENT ACTIVITIES

Provisions must be made for patient activities: there should be an individual assigned to this task.

Community resources should be made available, listed and utilized.

Religious services should be made available where possible.

A staff of visiting clergy of all faiths should be available and their services utilized.

Visiting hours should be available, listed, and made adequate for patients' desires but must also protect their conditions.

There should be an ample supply of equipment and material and supplies to provide for adequate patient activities.

CLINICAL RECORDS

Each patient must have a clinical record that includes the following:
    Identification and summary sheet
    Initial evaluation
    Authentication of hospital
    Physicians' orders
    Physicians' progress notes
    Nurses' notes
    Medication and treatment record
    Laboratory and X-ray reports
    Consultation reports
    Dental reports
    Social service notes
    Patient care referral reports
Medical records should be completed and maintained within the rules and regulations.

Storage of records should be done in accordance with state and local laws.

A qualifying medical record librarian consultant should be available.

TRANSFER AGREEMENT

There must be agreements with transferring facilities a reasonable distance from the nursing home.

Nursing homes and hospitals must agree on a transfer referral form.

If the facility has been refused a transfer in any instance, there must be written evidence of the refusal.

PHYSICAL ENVIRONMENT

Construction:

The facility must be structurally sound.

It must meet the construction codes and fire protection codes.

There should be no fire hazards in the facility.

It must comply with the fire inspector's reports.

It must have available the last inspection report from the fire department.

All hallways and doorways must be free from chairs or other things which would block patients' exit during fire.

Halls must have handrails.

Building must be fire resistant.

Electrical and Mechanical Systems:

All safety standards must be met.

All lighting levels must be met.

Standby emergency electrical system must be operational.

All hot water spigots must be kept under a temperature level of 110° F.

There must be a nursing call system.

There must be charting equipment.

Nursing Unit:

Adequate medication area must be present.

Utility room must be present.

The utility room kept clean and orderly.

Patients' Bedrooms:

Cubicles or curtains must be present in double and other multiple rooms.

Patients' doors must not have locks.

All patients' rooms must have access to the corridor.

All beds must have three feet between them.

Isolation Room:

Isolation room must be available.

Examination Room:

An examination room must be available.

Examination table must be present.

There must be adequate space for patient activities.

HOUSEKEEPING SERVICES

Housekeeping Personnel:
There must be a sufficient number of housekeeping personnel.
Cleaning done only by non-nursing personnel.
Free from obnoxious odors.
Storage area orderly with everything off the floor.

Linens:
Soiled linens handled only by one person from the bed to the laundry.
Clean linens stored neatly and covered when carried through the hallway.
Soiled linen in a bag when transported through the halls.

DISASTER PLAN

There must be a written procedure to be used in the event of disaster.
There must be a list of people to be notified in the event of disaster, as well as a floor plan showing location of signals, extinguishers and evacuation routes.
Fire drills must be conducted regularly.
The staff must be trained in fire and disaster procedures.
The fire plan must be posted.

UTILIZATION REVIEW PLAN

A utilization review plan approved by the state health department must be established.
At least two physicians must be members of utilization review committee.

INDEX

Page numbers in *italics* refer to tables and illustrations.

Absenteeism, of personnel, policies regarding, 5
Accidents, causative factors in, 227
    human element, 228
    involving patients, nursing responsibilities in, 33
    involving personnel, 6
      report of, *16*
    prevention of, 227–230
    types of, 230
Accounting, conventions of, 245
    management and, 244
    process of, 246
    system of, 246
      organization chart for, *260*
Accreditation, of facility, requirements for, 266–273
    and Medicare and Medicaid benefits, 266
Administration, of facility, 2
    and accreditation, 267
    organization chart for, *18*
    responsibilities of, and personnel policies, 5
Administrative consultant, qualifications and duties of, 3
Administrative physician, duties of, 4
    qualifications of, 3, 24
Administrative secretary, qualifications and duties of, 4
Administrator, of facility, requirements for, 2
Admission(s), check-off list for, *133*
    evaluation at, 128, *136–137*
    policies on, 24–25
    record of, 156
Aide, nurses', qualifications and duties of, 39
Alcohols, as disinfectants, 202
Ammonium compounds, quarternary, as disinfectants, 203
Antibiotics, record of, *145*
Arthropods, control of, 200
Assets, of extended care facility, 247
Autoclave, for moist heat sterilization, 194, 207
    temperatures and pressures attained in, *208*
Autopsy, 27
    permit for, *146*

Balance sheet, in accounting system, 251, *254*
Barber and beautician services, 236–238
    disinfection and sterilization of equipment in, 238
    facilities for, 236
    personnel for, 237
    use of chemical solutions in, 237
Bathing facilities, 193
Beautician services, 236–238
Bedbugs, control of, 199
Behavior, of patients, as safety factor, 229
Bland diets, *66, 68, 70, 72, 74, 76, 78*
Blankets, wool, washing formula for, *221*
Bleaches, in laundry washing, 220
Bruises, 46
Budget. See also *Accounting* and *Business services.*
    for nursing service, 32
Burns, 46, 230
Business services, 244–265
    accounting in, 245–254
    organization chart for, *244*

Capital, of extended care facility, 247
Cash receipt slip, *256*
Census reports, of facility, *161, 163*
Charge nurse, 29–30
    qualifications and duties of, 37–38
Charge ticket, for patient services, *255*
Chef, qualifications and duties of, 61
Children, diabetic diets for, *81, 83, 85, 87, 89, 91, 93*
Chlorine, as disinfectant, 202
Clinical records, 124–166. See also *Records, clinical.*
    and accreditation of facility, 271
Cockroaches, control of, 199
Communicable diseases, at facility, reporting of, 27
    patient care in, 42, 44

Community, resources of, for patient activities, 120
Conduct, standards of, for personnel, 6
Constipation, 47
Construction, of facility, and accreditation, 272
    and fire safety, 232
Consultant, administrative, of facility, 3
Consultant dietitian, qualifications and duties of, 60
Consultant pharmacist, qualifications and duties of, 112
Consultation, by occupational therapist, 105
Contamination, of food preparation areas, 54
Cook, qualifications and duties of, 62
Cooking, of foods, safety in, 57
Coronary attacks, 46
Crafts, 121

Daily assignment card, 44
Day room, 183
Death report, 146
Debits and credits, in accounting, system of, 248
Dental services, 113–114
    and accreditation of facility, 270
    implementation of program for, 114
Diabetic diets, 1200 calorie or 1500 calorie, 80, 82, 84, 86, 88, 90, 92
    1800 calorie or 2200 calorie, 81, 83, 85, 87, 89, 91, 93
Diabetic test record, 144
Diagnostic services, 113
    and accreditation of facility, 270
Diarrhea, acute, 46
Diet(s), adequacy of, 51
    modified, 66–93
        diabetic, 1200 calorie or 1500 calorie, 80, 82, 84, 86, 88, 90, 92
            1800 calorie or 2200 calorie, 81, 83, 85, 87, 89, 91, 93
        low fat, 1000 calorie, or 1000 mg. sodium, 67, 69, 71, 73, 75, 77, 79
        soft or bland, 66, 68, 70, 72, 74, 76, 78
    physician's request form for, 65
    therapeutic, 51
Dietary personnel, 50
    in-service education of, 63–64
    personal hygiene of, 51
    qualifications and duties of, 60–64
Dietary services, 50–93
    and accreditation of facility, 269
    characteristics of, 53
    food-borne disease in, control of, 53, 54
        equipment and, 56
        in menu planning, 54
    nursing responsibilities in, 31, 34
    purchasing in, 55
    supervision of, 50–51
Dietitian, 50
    consultant, qualifications and duties of, 60
Dining area, 183
Director of nurses, 29
    qualifications and duties of, 35
Disaster plan, 224–226. See also Emergency affecting facility.

Disaster plan (Continued)
    and accreditation of facility, 273
Discharge, of patients, check-off list for, 134
    physician's responsibility in, 26
    register for, 156
Disease, communicable, patient care in, 42, 44
    physicians' responsibilities regarding, 27
    food-borne, 53
Disease index, 157, 158
Dishwashing, procedures for, 59
Disinfectants, 201, 202–205
    factors governing effectiveness of, 205–207
Disinfection, equipment for, 194
    of barber and beautician equipment, 238
Doors, and fire prevention, 231

Earache, 46
Ectoparasites, control of, 199
Education, in-service, and accreditation of facility, 268
    for nursing personnel, 31, 48
Elevators, safety standards for, 188
Emergency, affecting facility, disaster plan for, 224–226
        and accreditation of facility, 273
        and water supply, 190, 225
        fire, procedure to follow in event of, 234
        heating system, 225
    and personnel injuries, 7
    in critically ill patient, 40, 45
    medications kit for, 111
    nursing responsibilities in, 33, 46
    pharmacy department drug tray for, 111
    physician's roles in, 26, 47
Employees. See also Personnel.
    applications for, 10–12
Environment, physical, of facility, 181–209
    recommended values for safety maintenance in, 184–188
Equipment, barber and beautician, 238
    for disinfection, 194
    housekeeping, 214–215
    nursing, 33
    physical therapy, 96, 98
Equity, owner's, statement of, in accounting system, 251, 253
Evaluation, admitting, of patient, 128, 136–137
Examination, physical, 128
    at admitting evaluation, 25, 137
    facilities for, 183
    post-mortem, 27
    permit for, 146
Exits, from facility, considerations for, 231
Expenses, in accounting procedures, 245, 247
Extended care facility, business services of, 244–265
    license for, 2
    physical aspects of, 181–209
        and accreditation, 272
        and construction materials, 232
        and fire safety, 231
    requirements for, 1–4
        federal, 1–2
Extinguishers, fire, 234, 235

Fainting, 46
Family, of patient, education of, 34
    privileges of, 23
Federal government, and Medicare act, 260–265
    requirements for extended care facility, 1–2
Finances. See *Accounting* and *Business services.*
Financial statement, in accounting system, 250
Fire, procedure to follow in event of, 234
Fire extinguishers, 234, *235*
Fire safety, 231–235
    automatic and mechanical controls for, 234
    regulations for, 233
Fleas, control of, 199
Flies, control of, 198
Flow chart, for clinical records, *126–127*
Food(s). See also *Diet(s)* and *Dietary services.*
    cooking of, 57
    holding of, following preparation, 57
    leftover, 54
    preparation of, 52
        and sanitary conditions, 52
    pre-preparing of, 57
    purchasing of, 55
    quality of, 51
    serving of, 58
    storage of, 56
Food-borne disease, 53
    thermal destruction and, 57
Food service. See *Dietary services.*
Food service worker, qualifications and duties of, 62
Formaldehyde, as disinfectant, 204
Frozen storage, of foods, 56
Drugs. See *Medications* and *Pharmaceuticals.*

Garbage, disposal of, 196, 197
Germicides. See also *Disinfectants* and *Sterilization.*
    in laundry washing, 220
Government, federal, reimbursement from, under Medicare, 260–265
    requirements for extended care facility, 1–2
Gratuities, to personnel, 7
Grooming, of personnel, 6

Hairdresser. See *Barber and beautician services.*
Headache, 46
Health, of personnel, 7
Health record. See also *Records, medical.*
    arrangement of, 153
    legal aspects of, 148–153
Hearing, disorders of, rehabilitation services for, 108
Heating, of facility, emergency in, 225
History, of patient, at admitting evaluation, 25, *136*
Holidays, religious, for personnel, 7
Home, nursing. See *Extended care facility.*

Housekeeping services, 210–215
    and accreditation of facility, 273
    and fire safety, 232
    equipment for, *214–215*
    in laundering area, 219
    measuring results of, 213
    personnel for, 210, 211
        tasks of, 212
    program for, considerations in, 210
Hygiene, personal, of staff, 6

Identification and summary sheet, for individual patient, *135*
Impaction, fecal, 47
Income statement, in accounting system, 251, *253*
Index, patient, 155, *158*
Indigestion, simple, 47
Infection report, *147*
Information, for personnel, posting of, 6
Injuries, accidental, of patients, 33
    of personnel, 6, 7
        report of, *16*
Insect control, 198–200
In-service education, and accreditation of facility, 268
    for nursing personnel, 31, 48
Insomnia, 46
Inspections, for fire safety, 233
Iodine, as disinfectant, 202
Isolation, facilities for, 183

Joint Commission on Accreditation of Hospitals, 266
Journal, for accounting data, 248, *252*
    payroll, 256, *258*

Kitchen, 189
    sanitation requirements for, 52

Laboratory services, 113
Lacerations, 46
Language, disorders of, rehabilitation services for, 108
Laundry, clean, finishing of, 222
    handling of, 217
    transporting of, 222
    soiled, assembly and sorting room for, 217
    handling of, 216
    sorting of, 219
    washing area for, 217
    washing of, formulas for, 220, *221*
Laundry services, 216–223
    facilities for, physical aspects of, 217
    personnel for, 219
    procedures for, 219–223
Lavatories, special plumbing fixtures for, 193
Laws, state, and accreditation of facility, 266
    compliance with, 2

Leave of absence, for patient, form for, 130
Ledger, for accounting data, 249
Ledger account, 253
  patient's, 255
Leftover foods, 54
Liabilities, of extended care facility, 247
Librarian, medical records, qualifications and
  duties of, 166
Lice, control of, 199
License, for facility, 2
  for staff, 2
Lighting levels, in facility, 189
Linen supply. See also Laundry services.
  daily requirements per bed, 223
  daily requirements per patient, 223
  maintenance of, 214
Lost and found, 8
Low fat diets, 67, 69, 71, 73, 75, 77, 79

Mail, to facility, 8
Management, administrative, of facility, 2–4.
    See also Administration.
  of business services, 244
Materials, nursing, 33
Mattresses, cleaning of, 222
Meals. See Diet(s) and Food(s).
Medical records. See also Records, clinical and
    Records, medical.
  advisory committee for, 20
  and accreditation of facility, 271
  nursing section of, 47
  physicians' responsibilities for, 27
Medical records librarian, qualifications and
  duties of, 166
Medicare, and accreditation of facility, 266
  cost determination for, methods of, 261, 262,
    264–265
  payment procedures for, 262, 263–265
  reimbursement to facility under, 260–265
Medications, charting of, 111
  dispensing of, 33, 109–114
  emergency kit of, 111, 111
  physicians' responsibilities in, 25–26
  stop orders for, 110, 129
Medications record, 132, 145
Medicines. See Medications and Pharmaceu-
    ticals.
Medicine cabinet, 110
Mentally disturbed patient, care of, 45
Menu(s). See also Diet(s).
  modified, 66–93
  planning of, 52
Mercurial compounds, as disinfectants, 203
Modified diets, 66–93

Narcotics, dispensing of, 109
  record of, rules and regulations for, 131
Nosebleed, 47
Nurse(s), charge, 29–30
  qualifications and duties of, 37–38
  director of, 29
    qualifications and duties of, 35
  in-service education for, 48–49

Nurse(s) (Continued)
  supervising, 29
    qualifications and duties of, 36–37
Nurses' aide, qualifications and duties of, 39–40
Nurses' notes, charting procedures for, 164–166
Nursing care plan, 31
  and accreditation of facility, 268
  forms for, 41, 42, 43
Nursing home. See Extended care facility.
Nursing services, and accreditation of facility,
    268
  and dietary supervision, 31
  emergency, 46–47
  of facility, organization of, 41
  policies on, 28–49
  purposes of, 28
  regular procedures of, 47
  restorative, 30
  24-hour, 30
Nursing unit, 30
  design of, 182
  secretary of, qualifications and duties of, 38
Nutrition. See also Diet(s).
  guides for, 51, 53

Occupational therapist, qualifications and duties of, 104–105
Occupational therapy, 100–107
  agreement form for, 106
  initial evaluation for, 101
    functional status chart for, 102–103
  treatment planning outline for, 107
Orderly, qualifications and duties of, 39–40
Orders, medications, 33, 129
  physicians' responsibilities in, 25–26
  physicians', 33, 129
Organization, of facility services, 18
Owner, of facility, and accreditation, 266
  and state law, 2

Patient, activities of. See Patient activities.
  bedroom of, 182
  behavior of, as safety factor, 229
  care of. See Patient care.
  critically ill, emergency in, 40, 45
    nursing responsibilities for, 40
  education of, 34
  long-term, and utilization review, 243
  mentally disturbed, care of, 45
  privileges of, 22–23
  rights of, to medical records, 151
  safety of, 181
  toilet facilities for, 182
    safety features of, 229
  transfer of, forms and agreements for, 167–180,
    168–170, 172–173, 176–180
Patient activities, 119–123
  and accreditation of facility, 271
  program for, areas and equipment for, 120
  goals of, 120
Patient care, daily assignment card for, 44
  in communicable disease, 42
    procedures for, 44

Patient care *(Continued)*
  in critical illness, 40, 45
  in facility emergency, 224
  policies of, 17–23
    and accreditation of facility, 267
    committee for, 18–22
    legal requirements of, 17
Patient status, changes of, facility policies regarding, 3
Payroll, journal for, 256, *258*
  taxes on, 256
Personnel, 3, 5–16
  and accreditation of facility, 267
  and fire safety, 232
  and utilization review, 243
  appearance and grooming of, 6
  attitude of, and accident prevention, 228
  conduct of, standards of, 6
  for barber and beautician services, 237
  housekeeping, 210, 211
  laundry, personal hygiene of, 219
  payroll of, 256, *258*
  promotion policies for, 8
  responsibilities of, 5–16
Pest control. See also *Insect control* and *Rodent control.*
  as housekeeping requirement, 213
Pharmaceuticals. See also *Medications.*
  dispensing of, 109–114
  storage of, 110
Pharmacist, consultant, qualifications and duties of, 112
Pharmacy, advisory committee for, 20
  and accreditation of facility, 270
  emergency drug tray of, 111, *111*
Pharmacy and therapeutics advisory committee, 20
Phenols, as disinfectants, 204
Physical examination, 128
  at admitting evaluation, 25, *137*
  facilities for, 183
Physical therapist, qualifications and duties of, 95, 97–100
Physical therapy, 94–97
  equipment and facilities for, 96, *98*
  non-professional assistant in, 95
  objectives of, 94
  physician's prescription for, 96, *99*
  reports and records of, 95
Physician, administrative, 24
    qualifications and duties of, 3–4
  attending, 24
  orders of, 33, 129
  prescription for physical therapy by, 96, *99*
  responsibility of, 24
  services of, and accreditation of facility, 267
  policies on, 24–27
Pillows, cleaning of, 222
Pine oil compounds, as disinfectants, 205
Plumbing system, of facility, 191
  special fixtures for, 193
Podiatric services, 114
Poisoning, 46, 230
Posting. See *Accounting.*
Post-mortem examination, 27
  permit for, *146*

Pregnancy, diabetic diets during, *81, 83, 85, 87, 89, 91, 93*
Program assessment advisory committee, 20
Progress notes, on individual patients, 129, *138, 139*
Promotion, of personnel, 8
Purchasing, of foods, 55
  and nursing service, 32

Receiving, of purchased foods, 56
Records, accounting, 244–265. See also *Accounting* and *Business services.*
  clinical, 124–166
    admitting evaluation, 128, *136–137*
    authorization for disclosure of, 148, *152, 153*
    confidentiality of, 125
    content of, 124
    death report, *146*
    filing systems for, 153–155
    identification and summary sheet, 125, *135*
    infection report, *147*
    legal aspects of, 148–153
    librarian for, 166
    narcotic record, 131
    nurses' notes, 164–166
    of medications, 132, *140, 145*
    ownership of, 149
    physicians' responsibilities for, 27
    principles for maintaining, 147–148
    procedures for handling of, *126–127*
    progress notes, 129
    quantitative review of, 128
    releases, 130
    retention of, 125
    staff responsibility for, 125
    temperature sheet, *141*
  index, of diseases, 157, *158*
    of patients, 155–157, *158*
  medical, advisory committee for, 20
    and accreditation of facility, 271
    and utilization review, 243
  nursing service, 32
  of utilization review, 243
  time and earnings, for personnel, 256, *257*
Recreation. See also *Patient activities.*
  director of, 122
    qualifications and duties of, 122
Rehabilitation, restorative services for, 30, 32, 94–108
Reminder form, *134*
Reports. See also *Records.*
  from nursing service personnel, 32
  special, of diagnostic laboratory tests, 130, *142–143, 144*
Restorative services, 94–108
  and accreditation of facility, 269
Revenue, in accounting procedures, 245, 247
Review, of patient's record, following admission, 128
  utilization, 21, 239–243
    and accreditation of facility, 273
    sample form for, *240–242*
Roaches, control of, 199
Rodent control, 200

Safety. See also *Accidents* and *Fire safety*.
  of patients, facility maintenance and, 181, *184–188*
  rules for, personnel and, 7
Salaries, of personnel, 8
  payroll journal and, 256, *258*
Sanitation, in food service operation, 52, 58, 60
  dishwashing and, 59
  evaluation of effectiveness of, 59
Secretary, administrative, qualifications and duties of, 4
  of nursing unit, qualifications and duties of, 38
Serving, of foods, 58
Sewage, disposal of, 192
Shifts, 9, *14–15*
Smoking, 232
Social Security Act, extended care facility requirements under, 1–2
Social services, 115–118
  and accreditation of facility, 270
  data obtained for, 115
Social worker, qualifications and duties of, 117
  consultant, 116
Soft diets, *66, 68, 70, 72, 74, 76, 78*
Solicitation, within facility, 6
Speech therapy, 107–108
Sprinkler system, for fire safety, 234
Staff. See also *Personnel*.
  licensing of, 2
State laws, and extended care facility, 2
  and accreditation, 266
  and ownership, 2
Statistics, on facility operation, calculation of, 157–161
  census reports for, *161, 163*
Stenographer, 4
Sterilization, agents of, 201
  equipment for, 194
  gas, 209
  methods of, 207–209
    dry heat, 208
      time-temperature relationships for, *209*
    moist heat, 207
      time-temperature relationships for, *208*
  of barber and beautician equipment, 238
Storage, of barber and beautician supplies, 237
  of clean laundry, 218
  of foods, chilled, 56
    dry, 57
    frozen, 56
Supervising nurse, 29
  qualifications and duties of, 36–37
Supplies, for nursing service, 33

Taxes, federal income, 256
  FICA, 257
  FUTA, 258
  payroll, 256, 260
Temperature sheet, *141*
Tests, laboratory facilities for, 113
  of physical therapy progress, 96, 99
Therapist, occupational, qualifications and duties of, 104–105
  non-professional physical, 95
  physical, qualifications and duties of, 95, 97–100

Therapy, occupational, 100–107
  agreement form for, *106*
  initial evaluation for, 101, *102–103*
  treatment planning outline for, *107*
  physical, 94–97
    equipment and facilities for, 96, *98*
    objectives of, 94
    physician's prescription for, 96, *99*
    reports and records of, 95
  speech, 107–108
Thermal destruction, of food-borne microorganisms, 57
Toilet fixtures, 194
Training, in-service, and fire safety, 232
  of dietary personnel, 63–64
  of nursing personnel, procedure for, 48
    skilled, 31
  programs of, 9
Transfer agreements, 167–180, *168–170*
  and accreditation of facility, 272
  community-wide, form for, *174–175*
  execution of, 170
  individual, forms for, *172–173, 176–180*
  legal requirements for, 171
  responsibility in, 170
Tray service, kitchen procedures for, 58
Treatment, occupational therapy, 100–107
  orders for, nursing responsibilities in, 34
    physicians' responsibilities in, 25–26
  physical therapy, 94–100
  plan for, *137*

Utilization review plan, 239–243
  and accreditation of facility, 273
  bases for, 242
  records for, 243
  responsibility for, 21, 239
  sample form for, *240–242*

Vacuum breakers, for waste disposal systems, 192
Vacuum cleaners, specifications for use of, *215*
Venomous insects, control of, 200
Ventilation, of laundry area, 218
Visitors, to patients, policies regarding, 23

Washers, dish, 59
  laundry, 217
Waste disposal system, of facility, 192
  handling procedures in, 194
  in barber or beauty shop area, 237
  typical wastes in, 196
Water supply, of facility, 190–194
  emergency in, 225
  hot, temperature ranges for, 191
Women, pregnant, diabetic diets for, *81, 83, 85, 87, 89, 91, 93*
Work sheet, for accounting data, 250, *259*
Working hours, 9, 13, *14–15*